D1483168

Politics, Science, and Dread Disease

Politics, Science, and Dread Disease

A Short History of United States
Medical Research Policy

Stephen P. Strickland

Harvard University Press   Cambridge, Massachusetts   1972

A Commonwealth Fund Book

This volume is published as part of a long-standing
cooperative program between Harvard University
Press and the Commonwealth Fund, a philanthropic
foundation, to encourage the publication of significant
scholarly books in medicine and health.

For T. G. S.

Contents

Preface

In his State of the Union Message of January 1971, President Richard M. Nixon urged the adoption of a new national goal— the conquest of cancer. To achieve that goal the President proposed a mobilization of scientific knowledge, professional expertise, and public funds, similar to the organized massive efforts of previous decades to build an atomic bomb and place a man on the moon. Thus, in one paragraph the President laid the predicate for a new national policy, if only by giving new momentum and greater specificity to one component of an old policy.

The federal government first began a cancer research program in 1922 when the U.S. Public Health Service established a Special Cancer Investigations Laboratory at Harvard University. That small effort stemmed from the interests and concerns of research scientists, including some in the employ of government. It remained so limited, even so obscure, an endeavor that members of the United States Senate only learned of it five years after its commencement.

Beginning in 1878, federal officials had from time to time expressly approved and encouraged other medical research efforts. In that year, serious epidemics of yellow fever and cholera caused Congress to enact the first federal quarantine law, which contained a provision for funds "for investigating the origins and causes of epidemic diseases." In 1912, this original research authority of the Public Health Service was expanded to include problems other than communicable diseases.

Before 1930, the national government's interest in medical research was spasmodic or otherwise limited. It was mainly manifested in the mounting of short-range efforts to meet short-term crises. In effect, there was no visible national policy on medical research, even as a component of a larger national policy on, or approach to, health or science. But in the two decades between 1930 and 1950 the contours of national policy in medical research took shape. In the next twenty years, medical research became one of the major components of the federal effort to promote the general welfare, and a large item in the federal budget.

In tracing the recent history of the medical research enterprise in the United States and the federal government's role in its development, I have attempted to illuminate the policy process, and to define and evaluate the specific policy involved, as well as to chronicle the sequence of fascinating scientific, organizational, and personal episodes that are the most obvious guideposts to that history.

For example, if the American people's hopes and fears about cancer begin to be answered by biomedical science in the next few years, future historians may identify President Nixon's initial call for a new attack against "the dread disease" as the keystone of a national policy which hastened the scientific breakthroughs. The President's speech is as convenient a historical marker as any in this continuing drama. But presidential specification of a desirable national goal is not tantamount to creation of a national policy. It is but one potent step in the process by which national policies are established or evolved.

Establishment of a policy of the kind President Nixon proposed and which the Congress in 1971 actually drafted involves setting up implementary machinery and ensuring an adequate supply of resources as well as choosing national goals. Policy making, therefore, most often requires agreement on both means and ends among those who have effective control over resources.

In the case of the new crusade against cancer, there could be no disagreement on the goal. But there was considerable difficulty in getting the agreement of Congress, which had traditionally led the way in developing national medical research policy, and of members of a critically important constituency, the biomedical science community, on how the crusade ought to be organized and under whose command, at what level it ought to be funded, and at what pace it ought to proceed. It took almost a year to achieve consensus on such issues despite the universal appeal of the basic idea.

The new policy-and-scientific assault on cancer was launched officially in December 1971, when the President signed the National Cancer Act. Another year has now passed, and some new research is underway, but the battle strategy—involving scientific, management, and purely political issues—continues to be shaped behind the lines.

All this is to suggest that policy making is a political process, although policy making and politics do not have interchangeable definitions. As I would define it, policy making is the process of deciding upon goals for the public good and delineating and activating strategies for attaining those goals. Policy making goes beyond that general activity aimed at resolving conflict over issues—one of the lowest common denominators among definitions of politics.

National policies need not, of course, always involve focused activity of the kind typified by the Manhattan Project or the space program. Policy can take the form of inactivity; it may, for example, involve nothing more than a conscious, collective attitude of "benign neglect" on the part of government toward an issue. (To be a *national* policy, however, such a posture would again require consensus; otherwise it would remain, say, merely a presidential policy.) National policies can also result from judicial interpretations of laws or constitutions, although, again, court decisions standing alone no more constitute policy than mere expression of presidential hopes or plans.

James L. Sundquist suggests that policies are simply strategies adopted by governments for the solution of problems.[1]

[1] Sundquist, *Politics and Policy: The Eisenhower, Kennedy, and Johnson Years* (Washington: Brookings Institution, 1968).

That is not to say that the adoption of problem-solving strategies is a simple matter for governments. On the contrary, as Charles E. Lindblom points out, policy making for democratic governments is so difficult a process that its salient characteristics are "complexity and disorder." [2] Yet policy making is as crucially important as it is inevitably difficult. As Sundquist says, "It is the capacity to make policy that is the basic dimension of the capacity to govern."

The complexity of the policy process in a democracy like ours relates not just to diversity of interest and hence to potentially conflicting goals among various segments of the populace. More specifically, it stems from our basic governmental arrangements whereby power is divided or shared. Thus, because government power is constitutionally divided, policy making is a shared activity. It is in fact so widely shared an activity that Lindblom would affix a permanent qualifier to the designation, "policy maker." There are only "proximate policy makers," he would argue. The national policy-making process involves many people, with the President at the head; in the ranks below him, many other public officials, including members of Congress and the cabinet and their advisers, have opportunities to affect policy decisions in critical ways. Yet no one of them, no matter where he sits, is in a position to "dictate" policy, to so control the process to the point of final action that he can claim exclusive authorship of a given policy.

In these circumstances, it should be expected that national policies often come into being gradually, incrementally, even disjointedly. If they evolve in such a way, rather than being established at one moment in time when specific consensus is achieved on a master plan, they are no less "policy" for that. Nor is it only small "policies" on unimportant issues that may evolve in that fashion, as the chapters that follow illustrate.

I should emphasize that those chapters do not simply make up a nice, academic policy study. Or at least that was not my

[2] Lindblom, *The Policy-Making Process* (Englewood Cliffs, New Jersey: Prentice-Hall, 1968).

intention. For the history of the medical research enterprise in the United States is first and foremost a story of a continuing, compelling quest, involving scientists, doctors, bureaucrats, lobbyists, and politicians—and reflecting the concerns of the people.

It may be readily and accurately imagined that in the several years this study has taken I have accumulated many debts to persons who were willing to help, at least by being willing to talk. Members and former members of Congress, the President's cabinet, and the White House staff; officials and former officials of the Public Health Service and the National Institutes of Health; and "members" of what it has become fashionable, and not at all inaccurate, to call the medical research lobby, have all been willing to share their views of policy making and particular "proximate policy makers," of medical research policy and its results, and of new and continuing medical research needs and opportunities. Their perspectives, gained in the course of scores of interviews, have greatly enriched this book. Their personal views have also made possible greater balance, and even greater accuracy, than would have been obtained had I stopped the research effort after completing the wide-ranging and detailed examination of printed documents.

Indeed, my list of those who made valuable contributions to this study is almost endless. I want to record my special and very deep gratitude to my wife, Tamara, and Sayers Brown, who were stalwart and imaginative research assistants. William H. D. Brown, Jr., Charles W. Johnson III, and David C. Pruitt III were always cheerfully willing to help me obtain original and secondary source materials. Dr. John F. Sherman, Deputy Director of the National Institutes of Health, was typically generous with his time, always being available to provide reactions to themes under development and to use his good offices to make access to key people and key documents easier for me. Mrs. Florence Stephenson Mahoney and Mrs. Albert D. Lasker answered many more questions than they really wanted to without ever making me feel that I was, in fact, imposing on them. Robert L. Peabody shared both scholarly knowledge and practical lessons from his own extensive experience in researching and writing about Congress and the policy process. He has been a true friend, as well as a more than competent adviser, throughout this endeavor. Terrance Keenan offered occasionally needed encouragement and consistently good counsel. And I am continually grateful to D. B. Hardeman for helping me secure the opportunity to begin the first part of this study nine years ago, for supplying many good ideas along the way, and for serving as a constant and delightful reminder of a most important fact—that government is people as well as structure and system. In addition to thanking each of these helpers, I must also absolve them, for they are neither necessarily responsible for, nor in agreement with, particular conclusions I came to and have reported in this volume.

Researching the subject presented here was a continuingly interesting and rewarding activity for me, even though the writing was a most difficult and demanding job, as it always is. I am grateful to have had the opportunity to do both. Therefore, I gladly record my gratitude to the Commonwealth Fund, my principal sponsor, and to the Ford Foundation and Mr. David Rockefeller for supplementary grants. Mr. Rockefeller's assistance is one more indication of his family's continuing interest in promoting activities that might directly or indirectly lead to the improvement of health.

I am always pleased and appreciative when my own bad typing is converted into clean, readable copy, and I thank Lillous Miller, Exa Murray, and my secretary, Zene Krogh, for performing that difficult task.

Though I feel no similar indebtedness, I am nonetheless gratified by the federal government's launching of a new national crusade to conquer cancer. It brings the story which begins in Chapter I of this study—an old story of scientists' long struggle with a persistent "enemy of man" and of public officials' recurring struggle with a difficult policy issue—full circle. I wish them success.

Politics, Science, and Dread Disease

I Conquering Cancer: The Origins of a National Policy

On May 18, 1928, in the Senate of the United States, the senior Senator from West Virginia, Matthew M. Neely, obtained the floor.

> Mr. President, the concluding chapter of *A Tale of Two Cities* contains a vivid description of the guillotine, the most efficacious mechanical destroyer of human life that brutal and blood-thirsty man has ever invented.
>
> But through all the years the victims of the guillotine have been limited to a few hundred thousands of the people of France.
>
> I propose to speak of a monster that is more insatiable than the guillotine; more destructive to life and health and happiness than the World War, more irresistible than the mightiest army that ever marched to battle; more terrifying than any other scourge that has ever threatened the existence of the human race. The monster of which I speak has infested and still infests every inhabited country; it has preyed and still preys upon every nation; it has fed and feasted and fattened . . . on the flesh and blood and brains and bones of men and women and children in every land. The sighs and sobs and shrieks that it has exhorted from perishing humanity would, if they were tangible things, make a mountain. The tears that it has wrung from weeping women's eyes would make an ocean. The blood that it has shed would redden every wave that rolls on every sea. The name of this loathsome, deadly and insatiate monster is "cancer".[1]

What Senator Neely wanted the Senate to do about cancer was to appropriate funds to conquer it. "Medical science," he pointed out, "has conquered yellow fever, diphtheria, typhoid, and smallpox" and "robbed leprosy and tuberculosis of their terrors . . . But in spite of all that physicians, surgeons, chemists, biologists, and all other scientists have done, cancer remains unconquered." [2]

A year earlier the Senator had favored a personalized assault on the dread disease, and had introduced a bill that would provide a $5 million reward "to the first person who discovered a practical and successful cure for cancer." The Senate had not actively considered that measure, but it attracted considerable publicity. Within a year Senator Neely had received some 2,500 letters from persons who claimed to possess infallible cancer cures. Their contents, said the Senator, had caused him to rethink the matter. Most of the letters, he said, were similar to that from Mrs. C. J., of Dayton, Ohio.

> Dear Sir: In reading the paper I saw a reward for the cure of cancer. Not that I am after the money, but just to show you what the Lord will do, I am sending an anointed handkerchief, and if you will do as I tell you, you will be cured of that disease. Now, just lay it over the cancer in the name of Jesus, and it is healed if you believe it. If this doesn't do any good, it is because you have no faith.[3]

Others variously prescribed arsenic, egg whites, soot from wood stoves, South African boggo, and stoneflower juice; but all they accomplished was to convince Senator Neely "that the plan to offer a reward for a cure for cancer set forth in my bill was imperfect, if not utterly futile." [4]

His revised plan, formulated in counsel with Dr. Joseph Bloodgood of Johns Hopkins University and others, was to have the Congress authorize the National Academy of Sciences "to investigate the cancer subject and report to Congress in what manner the federal government could assist in coordinating all cancer research and in conquering this most mysterious and destructive disease." The Senate Committee on Education and Labor unanimously approved the proposal and sent it to the Senate.[5]

Only one of Neely's colleagues, a fellow Democrat, disagreed with the plan: Senator Joseph Ransdell, sometime chairman of the Committee on Public Health and Quarantine. Ransdell, a dignified, goateed Louisianan, had become interested in public health in part because of the epidemics following floods of the Mississippi River; flood control was the principal cause he had championed in the Senate, although he attracted particular notice by advocating an amendment to the Constitution which would prohibit divorced persons from remarrying.[6] As often happens to congressional committee chairmen, Senator Ransdell's gradually developing knowledge of subjects under his jurisdiction seemed to bring with it genuine, if vested interest in those subjects. Specifically, he had become convinced that he could win fame by championing, along with flood control, public health measures. He had earlier introduced the bill establishing the first federal leprosarium. More recently, at the urging of Assistant Surgeon General Lewis R. Thompson, an early and ubiquitous in-house lobbyist for medical research, Ransdell had introduced a bill to establish the National Institute of Health— a move which transformed the old Hygienic Laboratory of the Public Health Service far beyond the change of name into the structure from which was to be launched a great national medical research enterprise.

At least one reviewer of history has suggested that the burgeoning of medical research in the United States in the post-World War II years was a direct and natural consequence of the careful planning and sophisticated strategy of those directing the government's relevant activities in an earlier period. Donald C. Swain states: "Their far-sighted policy, carefully calculated to advance the cause of federally sponsored medical research, made it possible for NIH to become the giant that it is today." [7] Swain mainly means the efforts of Public Health Service officials in the 1930's, and applied to that decade his judgment may be a fair one. But no farsighted, carefully calculated policy was in evidence in 1927 and 1928, when Neely first tried to interest the Congress in conquering cancer. Indeed, only Senator Ransdell seemed to know that the government was already supporting, and performing in its own laboratories, cancer research.

In 1922 the Public Health Service through its Division of Scientific Research had sponsored a small "cancer investigations laboratory" at Harvard Medical School. Simultaneously, scientists at the Hygienic Laboratory in Washington, D.C., had undertaken cancer research. For both the intra- and extra-mural cancer studies in that year, $11,000 was spent. It was projected that as much as $25,000 per annum might be needed later.[8]

Senator Neely first learned about these efforts when, subsequent to the Education and Labor Committee's unanimous endorsement of his 1928 plan, Senator Ransdell approached him and asked him to revise his bill (through amendment) so as to permit the Public Health Service to join with the National Academy of Sciences in carrying out the survey and making recommendations to Congress on how to proceed. Senator Neely, though apparently surprised, consented. "After familiarizing myself with its recent accomplishments . . . I became convinced that the Public Health Service should aid in making the investigation and report proposed in my bill." [9] The Senate adopted the amended measure without objection, authorizing $50,000 to accomplish the job.

Perhaps it is not unusual that only one Senator seemed to know in 1928 that the federal government was in any way or to any degree engaged in medical research. That effort, in the United States, had traditionally been left to the private sector while the government saw after other research concerns. In 1927, the year it ignored "the first bill that was ever offered in either house of Congress for the purpose of obtaining governmental assistance in solving the cancer problem," [10] Congress appropriated $10 million to eradicate the corn borer. In 1928, the year the Senate accepted the second Neely cancer bill, Congress had voted more than $5 million for the investigation of tuberculosis in animals. Indeed, said Senator Neely, the Congress had exhibited "unequaled liberality in protecting our domestic animals against every sort of disease and pest." [11]

In short, the federal government's support of research in the 1920's was not too far removed from its research support pattern and priorities of the 1880's: "Federal aid was extended in this period to the studies on the health of farm animals, while almost no funds were available for direct work on the diseases of man . . . This was partly because of the nature of medical science prior to 1885 and partly because human welfare brought no direct financial return. Hogs did." [12]

The private sector was not doing badly by medical research in 1928. John D. Rockefeller and his son John, Jr., had built up the Rockefeller Institute's endowment to $65 million by that year. The Institute had dispensed $20,000 in its first year, 1901, for medical research grants. In its second year, 1902, its budget was $1 million.[13]

In 1902 the federal government took a significant organizational step forward. The Marine Hospital Service became, when President Theodore Roosevelt signed the law, the Public Health and Marine Service of the United States. Its Hygienic Laboratory, begun at the Marine Hospital in Staten Island in 1887, was expanded from one division, bacteriology and pathology, to four, now including chemistry, pharmacology, and zoology. By specifying a system of communications among state and territorial health officers—for one thing, providing that the Surgeon General of the U.S. Public Health Service should convoke an annual meeting of such officers—the new law "legalized the supremacy of the Federal Government in the field of public health." [14] It also established a mechanism that was to become a

lasting central feature of the subsequent health research enterprise: an Advisory Board to the Hygienic Laboratory.

But if the government made organizational strides in 1902
that in retrospect seem commandingly important, its commitment to medical research was paltry compared to the commitment of private institutes. Its total budget for operating the
Hygienic Laboratory would not reach the $50,000 level until
1904.[15] The Rockefeller Institute alone was already spending
more than twenty times that amount.

The ratio of private-federal expenditures for medical research
continued relatively unchanged for the first four decades of the
century. And it was accepted as natural that the private side
should dominate; that the Rockefeller and Carnegie philantro-
pies, the Hooper, Cushing, Phipps, and Sprague Memorial Institutes, and the other private research organizations and private
foundations giving money for biomedical investigations, should
in effect constitute the national medical research effort. It could
even be said that the private sector was *expected* to support
medicine and medical research. Some other causes funded
privately—education and public welfare—were also the domain of public agencies, but medicine and biomedical research
generally were not. Thus it was that in 1940 "from the 63 foundations that contributed most for all purposes . . . medicine received about $9.5 million," more than any other activity; and a
sizeable although not easily identifiable portion of that was for
research.[16]

Delineations of public and private responsibility for the social
good in our country have mainly occurred for pragmatic reasons,
although they are often discussed in philosophical if not constitutional terms. Local responsibility and private initiative are
as strongly woven into the fabric of national values today as
they were in the early years of the Republic, even though national programs born of practical necessity (or of felt need)
suggest, in the aggregate, that most Americans accept the fed-

eral government's responsibility for the nation's welfare as being potentially all-pervasive.

Let a national need be obvious and the national government is considered to have authority to deal with it—even to deal with it directly, though without necessarily ignoring other options, and often using a combination of options by which it reduces its direct role to "partner" rather than dominant superior. Against such a background, those who wish to establish a new activity or policy direction involving a significant commitment of federal resources cast the need and the objective in national terms.

That cancer was a national problem which might require important, specific governmental action was not debated when Matt Neely asked the Senate to mandate a solution in 1928. The study he called for was a more cautious approach than a direct federal reward for a cure, but it presaged further, long-term federal commitment. After all, the cancer problem was "costing the United States almost $800 million a year, destroying more than a hundred thousand lives a year and inflicting more suffering and agony upon the American people than all the other diseases known to humanity." [17]

Nor did the fact that the private sector was working on the problem as part of its accepted, expected role in advancing the frontiers of good medicine and good health for the American people provoke any argument as to the right or need for federal involvement. Indeed, the Rockefeller Foundation—itself a symbol of private efforts and responsibilities in the premises— through its spokesman, Dr. Turner, encouraged the federal government's involvement via the plan offered by Senator Neely.[18]

The House of Representatives failed to act on the Neely bill after the Senate passed it in 1928. Senator Neely lost his re-election bid that fall,[19] and when his colleague Senator William J. Harris (D., Georgia) reintroduced the bill in 1929 it got nowhere. One reason may have been that, in the interim, the

Surgeon General of the Public Health Service, Dr. Hugh S. Cumming, convoked a conference on cancer to secure advice from interested scientists and others about what the PHS approach should be; the 17 persons who attended advised the Service to step up its efforts. The conference and knowledge of its conclusions gave the executive branch of government, through the PHS, the initiative—at least for the moment. It also gave the executive branch some planning time.[20]

Several decades later a visible, full-blown struggle developed between the executive and legislative branches over control of national medical research policy. The pattern of events in the 1920's and 1930's, with legislative moves and executive counter-moves over directions in medical research, suggest that a policy struggle was under way even then.

On the legislative side, Congress may have simply stumbled onto a good thing. Neely's original concern was no doubt as genuine as his original plan was naive. Further, to have the federal government mount a campaign to conquer cancer seemed liked a good idea—especially to politicians. To launch that crusade might bring fame, if not necessarily re-election. Senator Royal Copeland of New York, an M.D., former dean of the New York Flower Hospital and Medical School and former president of the New York State Board of Health, also pushed for action in the late twenties. The Senate's interest in cancer research was already recorded, and the Surgeon General's conference group had recommended an intensified effort. Why not, then, simply have the Congress appropriate more money for studies like those already in progress under PHS auspices? The Surgeon General replied that although he would be happy to have greater support for the PHS research efforts, he would prefer that any increase in funds not be limited to cancer research, but possibly used for broader, coordinated explorations of many disease problems.[21] The executive push was on.

On the same day that the Neely bill came up for discussion on the floor of the Senate in 1928, the Senate Commerce Com-

mittee favorably reported the bill introduced by Senator Ransdell but drafted by officials of the Public Health Service "to
establish and operate a national institute of health, create a
system of fellowships in said institute, and to authorize the government to accept donations for use in ascertaining the cause,
prevention and cure of disease affecting human beings, and for
other purposes." [22] Senator Ransdell was "delighted to know"
that his colleague from West Virginia was "striving so hard to
overcome the worst disease which we have in America today,
the awful disease of cancer." But while he was willing to go
along with the Neely cancer plan if the Public Health Service
were included, he did want to point out that his proposed "institute is not limited to any one disease, but takes in all the ills
that flesh is heir to." [23]

Of the two approaches offered for the Senate's consideration
at that juncture, there is no doubt which one the Public Health
Service preferred. Given PHS preferences, Senator Neely's subsequent defeat, Senator Ransdell's interest in pushing a bill that
was completely (so to speak) rather than partially (by means of
an amendment) his own, and Senator Copeland's understanding
of the scientific need for a broader approach, neither should
there have been any doubt which would ultimately become
law. It took two years, but the Ransdell Act was signed into
law on May 26, 1930. In addition to the features listed above,
it provided $750,000 for the erection of additional buildings to
house the research activity of the Public Health Service.[24] A
national policy on medical research was beginning to emerge.

The Ransdell Act could no more save its sponsor from defeat
by the phenomenon of Huey Long in the fall of 1930 than the
Neely bill had saved the West Virginia Senator from defeat in
1928. But having cooperated in guiding the PHS expansion plan
through the congressional maze, Ransdell was entitled to the
Service's gratitude. It was manifested in Surgeon General Cumming's appointment of the former Senator as chairman of the
newly created Conference Board on the National Institute of

Health, whose charge it was to consider how the new organization might properly and profitably be expanded. Also on the Board was the Senator's mentor and medical research guide, Assistant Surgeon General Lewis R. Thompson.

A counterproposal in time may save control. It did, for those directing the small federal medical research effort in the late twenties. The enterprise moved forward after the Ransdell Act of 1930, and the chief in-house lobbyist for that Act, Thompson, became Director of NIH while retaining his title as Assistant Surgeon General.

From the records available from that period, Thompson emerges as the most responsible figure behind what has become the most important vehicle for the performance of biomedical research in the world.[25] His sensitivity to congressional concerns and perceptions must have contributed to his decision that NIH must place increased emphasis on finding solutions to chronic diseases—a direction which caused considerable unhappiness among some NIH scientists and administrators. Further, Thompson was key to the successful effort to get Karl T. Compton, chairman of President Roosevelt's newly created Science Advisory Board, to appoint a special subcommittee on medical research. The subcommittee, including Dr. Thomas Parran, who was shortly to become Surgeon General, "recommended increased research in cancer, heart disease, tuberculosis, malaria, venereal disease, and dental problems." It also urged increased funds for "the scientific work of the Public Health Service."[26] As the next step "Thompson and his colleagues organized a letter-writing campaign to generate public and Congressional support for their cause. They pointed out that the prevention of disease tended to increase the economic security of the general population."[27]

The result of that and related efforts was the inclusion in Title VI of the Social Security Act of 1935 authorization of expenditures of up to $2 million annually for the "investigation of disease and problems of sanitation."[28] That provision, plus the appropriation of direct funds, caused the NIH budget to mount rapidly by standards then prevailing.

Meanwhile, Thompson had engineered an affirmative response to an offer, to the government, of land by a prominent Washington family, Mr. and Mrs. Luke I. Wilson, and ultimately secured a gift to the federal government of 82 acres in Bethesda on which to construct a major medical research campus.[29] With more funds, new and expanding facilities, and increased awareness—self-awareness, and awareness on the part of the public and their elected officials—the Public Health Service planned to go forward with a "program of attack on disease along some 70 lines." [30]

But it was really cancer that worried people most. And it was cancer that gave the people's elected representatives in Congress an easier handle on biomedical research. Some physician-researchers also thought greater attention should be given the cancer problem: Dr. Dudley Jackson of San Antonio, Texas, was one. He had done research on cancer for some years and received a grant for research on cancer from the National Institute of Health early in 1936. His efforts to find an answer through research, mighty though they may have been, were as nothing compared to his subsequent efforts to get the Congress to establish a "Central Government Cancer Committee," which would be a clearinghouse for information and would dispense grant funds and oversee research within the government.[31]

Dr. Jackson had little success in persuading top officials of the Institute and the Service of the desirability of such a cancer research scheme to narrow the focus while expanding support. Earlier, in 1930, he had failed to persuade Senator Hiram Johnson (R., Cal.), chairman of the Senate Commerce Committee, of the idea. The chance for realizing his goal came in the fall of 1936, when his friend Congressman Maury Maverick (D., Texas), just elected to a second term in Congress, agreed to introduce a bill to establish a national cancer institute. Dr. Jackson wrote to Dr. George McCoy, director of the Hygienic

Laboratory, on December 15, 1936, telling him of Maverick's agreement.[32]

Congressman Maverick also alerted the Public Health Service to his plan and asked for PHS suggestions and comments. He wanted to introduce a sound piece of legislation and he apparently discussed the matter with a number of persons. Mrs. Maverick recalls her husband saying that he had told President Roosevelt of his interest in having a special research effort for cancer, and that FDR advised that the easiest way to get special money for cancer was to tack on an amendment to the proposed appropriation for venereal disease control, then a popular health cause being funded in several millions of dollars annually.

The Surgeon General seemed to drag his feet in responding to Maverick. He was asked for counsel by Maverick around the first of the year but delayed a reply until April 6, 1937, when he sent the Texas Congressman several ideas for his bill. By that time Senator Hugh Bone, a Washington Democrat, had introduced his own bill to establish a cancer institute, having secured the signatures of all his Senate colleagues.[33]

The origins of the Bone bill are not as clear as those of the Maverick bill. There is no indication that Maverick knew that the Washington Senator was also preparing legislation, although the Public Health Service was certainly in consultation with Bone, too. A political associate and sometime campaign manager of Senator Bone, Saul Haas, claims to have interested Bone in the idea; and he helped secure the support of all other Senators. Only one of Bone's colleagues balked, on the grounds that direct federal involvement in cancer research "was a step toward socialized medicine." When his wife developed cancer he withdrew his opposition and became the ninety-sixth signatory to the bill.[34]

The Bone bill was introduced in early April 1937 and the Maverick bill on April 29. Twenty-six other House members joined Maverick in sponsoring it. Meanwhile, Senator Bone had gotten his young colleague from Washington, freshman Representative Warren Magnuson, to introduce a bill identical to his Senate measure.

When the Bone bill was sent to the Senate Commerce Committee the chairman, Senator Royal Copeland, asked the Surgeon General for some help. He wrote: "When a bill which is of special interest to one of the Departments is under consideration by a Congressional committee, it is customary to have somebody from the Department in question assigned to do the 'legwork.' I wish you would assign somebody from your staff to consult with me frequently about the steps taken to have a hearing and prepare the argument in favor of the bill." [35]

Outside pressure—almost a Conquer Cancer Crusade—had been building up. No doubt it had much to do with the entire Senate's endorsement of the Bone bill. The medical section of the American Association for the Advancement of Science had deliberated on the subject at its December 1936 meeting. Reporting and elaborating on the focus of that meeting, *Fortune Magazine* carried an article on its March 1937 issue entitled "Cancer, the Great Darkness." *Life* and *Time* also gave prominent notice to the subject in that period, and a wave of letters swept into congressional offices.[36]

If the pressure exerted on Congress, partially generated by those with special interest in the legislation in question, was not unusual in the history of our legislative process, the Congress' reaction certainly was. In an extraordinary move, joint Senate-House hearings were held on all the bills that had been introduced, on July 8, 1937. A compromise bill was enacted on July 23, and the National Cancer Institute Act became law upon the President's signature on August 5.[37]

Events had moved so swiftly that the executive branch reports were not submitted until after the congressional hearings had commenced.[38] The President's desire not to have authorized more than $1 million annually for research on cancer was honored (an annual authorization of $700,000 was finally approved);[39] but the Public Health Service's opposition to an advisory council on cancer was over-ridden, and such a council was given authority to review all research projects and certify its approval of them prior to their funding by the Surgeon General.[40]

The National Cancer Institute was authorized to conduct and foster research and studies relating to the cause, prevention, and methods of diagnosis and treatment of cancer; to promote the coordination of cancer research; to provide fellowships in the Institute (later amended to include institutions outside the government); to secure counsel and advice from cancer experts from the United States and abroad; and to cooperate with state health agencies in the prevention, control, and eradication of cancer.[41]

The American Society for Control of Cancer supported the bill, including the provision establishing an advisory council. The American Medical Association was dubious. Such an institute could turn out to be a forerunner of others, suggested AMA spokesman Dr. Olin West; and he didn't think that was a very good idea.[42] The AMA *Journal* warned: "The danger of putting the government in the dominant position in relation to medical research is apparent." [43]

Chairman Royal Copeland, on the other hand, thought it might be well to extend the idea. Other Senators, including Senator Robert LaFollette of Wisconsin, immediately went to work "on measures designed to create institutes for other medical research problems." [44]

Dr. James Ewing, a prominent physician-scientist of the day, evidenced still another attitude which was to recur throughout the history of NIH and the national medical research enterprise. He accepted membership on the National Cancer Advisory Council but he was skeptical of the whole approach: "This solution [to cancer] will come when science is ready for it and cannot be hastened by pouring sums of money into the effort." [45]

II   The War Years and Reconversion:
Hazards and Possibilities

During World War II the government had, for once, a clear, direct, purposeful medical research policy. And it had a centralized system, a strong organizational mechanism for effectuating it.

The National Defense Research Committee, created by President Roosevelt in 1940, quickly proved the efficacy of a coordinated approach to weapons development. The President consequently decided to create a comparable committee to force a coordinated approach in military medicine—an approach and program on which, up to that time, the several military services and the Public Health Service had not been able to agree. In July 1941 the Office of Scientific Research and Development, with parallel committees in medicine (CMR) and weapons (NDRC), was created by executive order and placed under the direction of Dr. Vannevar Bush, president of the Carnegie Institution, who already headed NDRC.[1] Dr. Bush suggested that the President appoint as chairman of CMR Dr. A. N. Richards, who was Vice President for Medical Affairs of the University of Pennsylvania.

Also named to the Committee on Medical Research were representatives from the Army, Navy, and Public Health Service and distinguished scientists and medical administrators from outside government. Dr. Lewis Weed, dean of the Johns Hopkins Medical School and chairman of the Division of Medicine of the National Research Council, was designated vice chairman of the Committee; the others were Dr. A. Baird Hastings of Harvard, Dr. A. R. Dochez of Columbia, Col. J. S. Simmons (later promoted to Brigadier General) of the Army Surgeon

General's office, Rear Admiral Harold W. Smith of the Navy's Bureau of Medicine and Surgery, and Assistant Surgeon General of the Public Health Service L. R. Thompson. A year later Dr. Thompson was replaced by Dr. Rolla E. Dyer, who had become Director of the National Institute of Health.[2]

The Committee on Medical Research had the job of "mobilizing the medical and scientific personnel of the nation . . . recommending to the Director [of OSRD] the need for and the character of the contracts to be entered into with universities, hospitals, and other agencies conducting medical research activities, and submitting recommendations with respect to the adequacy, progress and results of research on medical problems related to the national defense."[3] In short, CMR's job was to create and oversee a major program of medical research aimed at reducing the effects of disease and injury stemming from military action or relating to the national defense.

To accomplish that job CMR organized, with the help of the National Academy of Sciences—National Research Council, 51 committees and panels to review program needs in many fields; ultimately let 593 contracts with 135 universities, hospitals, research institutions, and industrial firms; and utilized the services of approximately 1,700 doctors of medicine and 3,800 scientists and technologists. Between 1941 and 1947, CMR spent $25 million through its six divisions: Medicine, $3.8 million; Surgery, $2.8 million; Aviation Medicine, $2.4 million; Physiology, $3.9 million; Chemistry, $2.3 million; and Malaria, $5.6 million.[4] "Never before," Dr. Richards later said, "has there been so great a coordination of medical scientific labor."[5]

Operating under a direct presidential mandate, with a clear purpose and what was tantamount to a blank check, the Committee's success in achieving policy goals can be measured in part by specific research results in medicine. The development and wide use of penicillin, sulfonamides, gamma globulin, adrenal steroids, and cortisone, among other drugs and techniques, saved hundreds of thousands of lives during the war itself and many millions more in the postwar period when they were applied to civilian use.

Congress was impressed. It attributed the "magnificent progress" in medical research to "adequate financing, coordination and teamwork." [6] And particularly impressive to some Congressmen was how "adequate financing" could speed up conquest of disease and medical problems. Dr. Richards reported to a fascinated Senate committee on a breakthrough in blood plasma by

> one of the most productive and interesting of the groups we have had the privilege of financing . . . Now, that investigation was started at Harvard University, with support of the Rockefeller Foundation, back in 1938, and has been continued up to the present. The amount of money assigned to it [previously] was $14,000, whereas, in the continuation of the work during the past three years we have spent over half a million . . . At the beginning, it was on the laboratory scale, wholly, and the products were curiosities. Now the products are commercially available and being supplied, or are ready to be supplied, in huge quantities.[7]

Dr. Chester Keefer, CMR's medical administrative officer, reported a similar life-saving speedup in the development of penicillin: "When one reflects upon the fact that it was only 30 months ago that the first patient was treated adequately in this country [with penicillin] and that now we have enough material to meet military needs and a moderate supply for civilians, it is a source of satisfaction. It is the finest example of what can be accomplished by collaborative efforts in the medical sciences when the proper leadership and cooperation are available."

Committee Counsel: "Dr. Keefer, would you be able to hazard a guess . . . as to when the development of penicillin might have reached this present stage if it had not been for this cooperative effort which you spoke of, under the OSRD? . . . it is perhaps safe to assume that it would have been a number of years at least."

Dr. Keefer: "I believe that is a safe statement, yes."

Committee Counsel: "And that, of course, would mean not only many more deaths and continued disabilities among the soldiers, but it would also mean a great many more deaths and disabilities among the civilian population."

Dr. Keefer: "That is a correct statement." [8]

By 1944, with the Allied Forces making steady progress in Europe, top officials began thinking about postwar planning on many fronts. Not long after its third birthday, in July 1944, the Committee on Medical Research was instructed by Dr. Bush to "make plans to facilitate the gradual transition of its program into peacetime arrangements when the appropriate time arrives." [9] At the request of the Secretaries of War and Navy, the President of the National Academy of Sciences (now Dr. Lewis Weed, vice chairman of the CMR) established the Research Board for National Security in November 1944; one of its purposes was to plan for postwar research.

Dr. Bush himself was working on a plan for continuing in peacetime the highly successful collaboration between government and the private sector, especially the universities, in research. President Roosevelt had asked Bush for recommendations on the subject, evidencing in his request a special interest in medical research; referring to the "war of science against disease," he cited as a particular concern the fact that the annual death rates in the United States from one or two diseases were higher than those on the battlefields.[10]

Meanwhile, in 1943, the Surgeon General of the Public Health Service, Dr. Thomas Parran, appointed a committee of three (including a young PHS officer who was to replace Parran as Surgeon General, Leonard Scheele) to make recommendations for the reorganization of PHS so as to better equip it to operate in the future. The in-house recommendations led to a legislative proposal to revise and consolidate all statutes under which PHS operated. Signed by the President on July 1, the Public Health Service Act of 1944 gave the Service authority similar to that assigned to the Committee on Medical Research at the start of the war: "to pay for research to be performed by universities, hospitals, laboratories, and other public or private institutions." [11] It was to support such research through grants, rather than contracts; and it was given specific authority to give grants to individuals. The main change, suggested one observer, was that in the new law Cangress "crossed out 'cancer' and inserted 'medical'." It seemed a small change and at the time was scarcely noticed, like a yet undetected pregnancy.

Congress was, at that point, giving more attention to the larger picture. In 1944 hearings that presaged some of the most important health legislation ever to be proposed and in part enacted, Senator Claude Pepper's Subcommittee on Wartime Health and Education, explored every aspect of that broad field. Particularly disturbed by Selective Service reports that approximately one-third of the men examined for induction into the military during the war were physically or mentally unfit, Pepper subsequently focused hard on the relation of research to the nation's health.[12] He thought that "it would be a wise expenditure of public funds to aid medical research and that the expenditure of more funds in medical research would lead to a longer life and better health for the people of the country." [13]

Despite the thought and planning on postwar medical research policy begun in 1944 or earlier, no clear policy had been formulated by the war's end. Nor was a long-term research policy to be settled in anything like the way wartime policy and program direction had been established.

As he pondered the future of government support of research, Dr. Bush came to favor a unified approach, to be manifested in the creation of a National Science Foundation which would insure a coordinated approach to all the nation's research needs and would simultaneously insure against government interference in the conduct of such research in the private sector. But the committee Dr. Bush had appointed, under Dr. Walter W. Palmer, to make recommendations specifically about the continuation of government-sponsored medical research, proposed at first that "the Federal agency concerned with medical research could be created *de novo* and be independent of all existing agencies." [14]

Bush used the Palmer Committee report in such a way that its recommendations did not contradict his plan for a National Science Foundation; yet Bush himself, according to Dr. Parran, had suggested earlier that when the Committee on Medical Research went out of business at the end of the war, the Public Health Service would be the natural agency to take over most of the uncompleted research projects and the unexpended funds.

Senator Pepper had been asked in 1944 by Dr. Ross McIntyre, the President's physician, not to hold hearings on the question of a special medical research agency. The compromise was that the hearings would go forward but that no recommendations would be made pending the report Dr. Bush was preparing. Pepper concluded his hearings in December 1944, saying that the Committee "will be recessed until further call, which will be, as I said, after we get access to the report of Dr. Bush, at which time we hope to proceed further with the actual formulation of legislation leading to the establishment of some proper national research agency, through which may be channeled Federal funds for the encouragement of research in the medical field." [15]

The Committee's January report merely states that it was essential "for the Federal Government to provide the resources for coordinated attack on medical problems which affect the country as a whole." [16]

When Vannevar Bush's report to the President, *Science, The Endless Frontier,* emerged in July 1945, its proposal of a national science foundation was introduced in Congress by Senator Warren Magnuson. Many of Magnuson's colleagues were dubious, feeling that what was being proposed was an elitist scientific establishment, funded by Government but operated exclusively by and for researchers. Doubts on the part of scientists about the propriety and safety of political direction of such an agency, and doubts on the part of the top public officials, including the President, as to the wisdom and propriety of creating a public agency over which there would be little public control, were factors which delayed the creation of a federal science agency for five years.[17] And that delay invited the evolution of quite a different approach to any program for medical research.

The American Medical Association had agreed to support creation of a science foundation—the work of OSRD during the war having demonstrated, said Dr. Morris Fishbein, "that federal funds could be used satisfactorily to promote research and speed medical discoveries." But he warned that "the foundation must avoid bureaucratic domination of research" and restrictions on research scientists.[18] At a meeting in Pittsburgh in October 1945, AMA officials agreed on such a position; but they informed Senator Magnuson that any significant departures from the bill he had introduced, or any serious delay in its passage, might cause them to change their position and campaign for a separate foundation.[19] Senator Pepper was another who had agreed to support the NSF approach, rather than work for the separate National Medical Research Foundation which he had once contemplated; but despite lending his name to the proposed NSF legislation, his strongest interest was in the medical field.

Tentativeness and uncertainty were reflected in all approaches to national postwar research policy. Even the President himself seemed unclear or undecided about key features of any plan under which government would continue its support of private scientific exploration. In September 1945, following the surrender of Japan, President Truman sent a special message to Congress presenting a 21-point program for conversion to peacetime. In it he urged the early adoption of legislation for the establishment of a single research agency which would discharge the following functions:

1. Promote and support fundamental research and development projects in all matters pertaining to the defense and security of the Nation.
2. Promote and support research in the basic sciences and in the social sciences.
3. Promote and support research in medicine, public health, and allied fields.
4. Provide financial assistance in the form of scholarships and grants for young men and women of proven scientific ability.
5. Coordinate and control diverse scientific activities now conducted by the several departments and agencies of the Federal Government.
6. Make fully, freely, and publicly available to commerce, industry, and academic institutions, the fruits of research financed by Federal funds.[20]

He reiterated his belief about "the desirability of centralizing these functions in a single agency" and asked the Office of Scientific Research and Development and also the Research Board for National Security to continue their work until the Congress acted on his request.[21]

Two months later, in his special message on health, the President took a somewhat different tack; but he reconciled his new emphasis on support for medical research by various federal agencies with his earlier message:

In my message to the Congress of September 6, 1945, I made various recommendations for a general Federal research program. Medical research—dealing with the broad fields of physical and mental illnesses—should be made effective in part through that general program and in part through specific provisions within the scope of a national health program.

Federal aid to promote and support research in medicine, public health and allied fields is an essential part of a general research program. Federal aid for medical research and education is also an essential part of any national health program . . . Coordination of the two programs is obviously necessary to assure efficient use of Federal funds.[22]

Wartime unity of purpose and agreement on means had evaporated. The effort to establish a clear, comprehensive national research policy was marked, for several years beginning in 1944, by shifting attitudes and conflicting proposals—and no action. Into the policy gap stepped the Public Health Service.

When called to testify on the proposed National Science Foundation bill in 1945, the spokesman for the Public Health Service, Dr. Rolla E. Dyer, avoided saying whether he was for or against the measure. He pointed out that the Public Health Service already had (especially since the statutory revisions of the previous year) "all of the authority in reference to health and medical research that is contemplated for the proposed foundation." And he admitted his concern about "preserving the scientific integrity and independence of [his] organization," just as the head of any similar enterprise would be concerned.[23]

Meanwhile, apparently following up conversations between Surgeon General Parran and Dr. Bush, Dr. Dyer had written to Dr. Richards as early as August 1944 (one month after CMR had been given sufficient legislative authority on which such a request could be based) suggesting that the Committee on Medical Research contracts be continued, when CMR closed shop, by the Public Health Service.[24] The Bureau of the Budget had opposed the provision of new funds to match the new research grant authority, but it did not mind the simple transfer of funds, represented by contracts in force, from CMR to PHS.[25]

The concept is abroad today as in the past that the legislative process is a matter of executive initiatives and congressional reactions: The President proposes and the Congress disposes; Government policies are initially worked out within the executive decision-making apparatus and, where necessary, are submitted to the legislative branch for ratification, or modification, or rejection. It is difficult to adduce evidence that this is *not* the way things generally work, even though a number of political scientists have, through illustrations of policy initiatives and program formulation that have come about in other ways, sought to establish a case for extraexecutive policy making.[26] Most observers will agree that the policy process is somewhat circular, with the real origin of a policy—or a thought or idea that becomes policy—a most elusive matter. Nor, perhaps, is it really important who got the idea first, or who is entitled to most credit for policy successes or most blame for policies that are unproductive or otherwise unsuccessful.

It is nonetheless informative, and important, to recognize that what have sometimes been considered as policy initiatives by the executive are in fact specific reactions to proposals of legislators. President Roosevelt's request to Vannevar Bush to formulate a policy and mechanism for government support of science and research after World War II, and Bush's subsequent policy proposal, were in part the result of Bush's alarm at features of a plan already being advanced: that of Democratic Senator Harley Kilgore of West Virginia.[27]

Similarly, actions and decisions which on the surface seem to indicate foresight, initiative, and even empire building on the part of bureaucrats may instead have to do with another bureaucratic trait—desire to protect existing domains. Surgeon General Thomas Parran and Assistant Surgeon General L. R. Thompson may have written the language of the National Cancer Act, and thereby preserved authority for the Public Health Service over it; but they did not really favor the idea of a separate cancer institute at first and got involved in influencing the outcome of the legislative initiative only when it was clear that *some* cancer bill *would* be enacted. And, although Public Health Service officials were involved in drafting the language of the Ransdell Act which created the National Institute of Health in 1930 (and although "Jimmy" Thompson helped Senator Ransdell guide that bill through the congressional as well as the executive maze), there was real reluctance on the part of a number of senior PHS officials to see any change at all. Memoranda from several of them on the first Ransdell bill to create a National Institute of Health indicate opposition to any new feature but larger appropriations; and even after admitting that the PHS research activity could and perhaps should be stepped up, they invariably cautioned against "growth of a mushroom type." [28]

Dr. A. M. Stimson, an assistant surgeon general, thought it "questionable whether there is any need for a new institution to be known as the National Institute of Health . . . It would seem therefore more in line with the best principles of legislation to make possible the carrying out of enlarged activities by larger appropriations, rather than by the establishment of a new institute." Even so, "the proposal for greatly enlarged appropriations for public health research work is subject to qualification." [29] Dr. George McCoy, director of the Hygienic Laboratory, was especially concerned lest the name of his organization be changed; "on the whole, after having studied [the bill] quite thoroughly," he saw "no material advantage from its enactment into law," although he thought its disadvantages might be overcome "by suitable amendments." [30] Dr. Dyer was in any case impressed with the "evidence of public sentiment" that "the Government should take a more active part in medical progress than it has in the past." [31]

Of particular concern to Dr. McCoy and other senior scientists and administrators was a provision allowing the Surgeon General to accept private contributions for the research effort. That, by the report of one observer close to Dr. McCoy, constituted a very serious threat indeed. "In addition to the possibility that the money will be expended for futile and useless purposes, there is also the danger that alien interests will secure an unwarranted influence on the administration of the institute . . . it may constitute an entering wedge, and for these reasons it is not viewed favorably by many of the older commissioned officers at the institute." [32]

Although the Public Health Service participated, in the end, in drafting and securing passage of the Ransdell Act, PHS (or at least many of its leaders) would much rather have been simply left alone—a sentiment which often recurred, if indeed it did not consistently dominate.

None of this is to deny the possibility of foresight, or prescience, on the part of bureaucrats. It is possible that the Public Health Service—National Institute of Health's purposeful movements to fill the policy vacuum of 1945–46 were based squarely on those qualities, and on a conscious, calculated plan to have NIH become the most important medical research institution in the world. The Surgeon General had, after all, some years earlier (1935) specified 70 research areas that NIH would have liked to explore if it but had the funds and the authority. And in his assessment of postwar medical research needs, Dr. Parran called for "new programs to emerge from the blueprint stage," stressing mental illness, heart disease, and chronic diseases of old age.[33]

But the uncharacteristically quick steps taken by PHS-NIH to secure most of the remaining wartime contracts from the Committee on Medical Research seemed more like defensive than offensive tactics. If ambivalence and contradiction marked the various proposals designed to establish a clear national research policy, including medical research policy, no one, in any case, was pushing PHS-NIH as the instrument for attaining policy goals except PHS-NIH. Bush wanted medical research to be a part of the National Science Foundation's business; Dr. Palmer wanted a brand new agency, patterned after Great Britain's Medical Research Committee. And Chairman Pepper, in evaluating the present and praising the past while looking to the future, seemed to ignore the government's existing medical research agency as he opened his 1944 hearings. "The record of accomplishment," he said, "rests solidly on the high achievements of medical science before the war. It has been made possible by the patriotic service of the universities, the scientific societies, the National Research Council, and most of all, by the scientists themselves." [34]

The Public Health Service—National Institute of Health must have felt left out and vulnerable. The Institute's budget the two years immediately preceding the war (fiscal 1940 and 1941), had been only slightly over $700,000, with less than a third of that awarded in research grants. (Private foundations in 1940 gave $4.7 million for research on medical problems.) During the war years, although the total appropriation for NIH began to grow, grant money—the stuff on which constituencies can be built—declined.

Based on Palmer Committee estimates, Dr. Bush suggested in 1945 that "the amount which can be effectively spent for medical research in the first year [of a postwar program] should not exceed $5 million" and that "after a program is effectively underway perhaps 20 million dollars can be spent effectively";[35] others suggested that, "as quickly as possible, national expenditures for medical research should reach $300 million annually." [36] In that year (fiscal 1946) NIH spent $850,000 for grants, and its total appropriation was approximately $3 million. To protect its status as the federal government's ongoing medical research agency, NIH very much needed to expand and become more visible.

If, then, the Public Health Service could secure the transfer of a significant number of wartime research contracts to NIH, its position would be more secure. There was one serious problem in the tactically bold, strategically conservative plan: the microbiologists who had traditionally constituted the PHS research teams and epitomized NIH research interests were disturbed that *contracts* under which scientists were performing *applied research* in *specific efforts* to reduce the effects of *particular diseases* were to be taken over by NIH. The same attitude that abounded in the Hygienic Laboratory in 1930, regarding acceptance of funds from outside the regular government channels for research, recurred when the possibility of NIH securing wartime applied research contracts developed.

The problem could be said to relate to the language of the 1930 Act itself. Funds were to be expended "for study, investigation and research in the fundamental problems of the diseases of man." [37] Though some, especially political figures, always stressed "diseases of man," others, especially working scientists, inevitably emphasized "fundamental problems."

There was no denying that the wartime research contracts were specifically focused on "military medical problems." But Dr. Dyer recommended in his formal suggestion to chairman Richards of the Medical Research Committee that NIH had both authority and interest in assuming jurisdiction of the contracts remaining and that, for the sake of the nation's future (in war as well as in peace, for he thought another war might come), not only should the "promising projects now underway" be continued, but "further research on the disease of man of non-military as well as military importance should be undertaken." [38] Dyer, according to persons who worked with him, was no mean diplomat; he could, they say, project the image of the cautious, conservative scientist, vis-à-vis his professional peers, while stretching administrative powers and statutory authority to new lengths in dealings with the world outside NIH. The objective at hand was beefing up the NIH status as a major governmental research institution; especially given the Bureau of the Budget's reluctance to commit new funds, the easiest way to do that was to get CMR's contracts. Reconciling the kind of research those contracts represented with the kind traditionally undertaken by NIH scientists and favored by the older Public Health Service officers could come later. For the time being the agency must expand in order to survive.

In January 1946 the Committee on Medical Research of the Office of Scientific Research and Development met for a final series of important meetings. Although it did not formally expire until the following year, its wartime mission was accomplished.

Dr. A. N. Richards, who had presided over the dispensation of $25 million during the life of the Committee, now presided over distribution of the remaining contracts. Of the seven members of the Committee, only the chairman and the three government representatives participated in the immediate decisions; the three were Admiral Smith of the Navy, General Simmons of the Army, and Dr. Dyer, assistant surgeon general of the Public Health Service and director of the National Institute of Health. A member of the Committee on Medical Research recalled the process.

> We went right through them one by one . . . Dr. Richards would say, "General Simmons . . . does the Army want this contract?" "No." Then he would say, "Admiral Smith, does the Navy want this contract?" And Admiral Smith would say no to all of them, one by one, because he knew they were in the process of developing ONR [Office of Naval Research]. That was going to be their program, which was not yet underway . . . So then he would say "Dr. Dyer, do you want this program?" And he said "yes." So by the time we got through, Dr. Dyer had almost all of them.

The significance of the transfer is most easily seen in dollar terms. From an expenditure of $180,000 for research projects in fiscal 1945, the figure went to $850,000 for fiscal 1946 and in 1947, the year most of the contracts were transferred, to $4 million. With its new statutory authority, and its new contracts, the agency needed more manpower and a bigger administrative budget. So in the same year, calendar 1946, the Congress appropriated for NIH for fiscal 1947 almost $8 million—more than a tenfold increase since the start of the war and almost four times what its budget had been when the Japanese surrendered to General MacArthur in August 1945.[39]

Whatever course the government ultimately chose for its peacetime research support, the National Institute of Health could no longer be overlooked.

As for the potential dilemma involving, on the one hand, Congress' desire to have NIH continue producing victories in the war against disease as the OSRD had done during the war and, on the other, microbiologists of the Public Health Service, and scientists now back in their university laboratories who were damned if they'd allow interference with their freedom and pet research efforts, NIH spokesmen produced a calming rationale:

> Although the Public Health Service awarded a few grants for cancer research every year from 1937 on, the broad program began in 1946 with the transfer of 50 projects from the Office of Scientific Research and Development when that agency was dissolved. The new program had as its objective the improvement of the nation's health through the acquisition of knowledge in all the sciences related to health. In the sense that the new knowledge is sought for the purpose of improving health this program is one of applied research, but many of the grantees consider their projects basic. Those who established the program believed that the maximum progress can be achieved only if scientists enjoy freedom to experiment without direction or interference, and they drew up the policies and procedures accordingly . . . Congress imposes a degree of control and direction when it appropriates funds earmarked for research on a designated disease or specific organ . . . In actual

practice, however, it has been possible to provide reasonably equal opportunity for scientists regardless of their specialty in the health field, since the earmarked areas are broad and overlap to a considerable degree, especially with regard to basic medical sciences.[40]

III   The Rise of the Research Lobby:

A New Mobilization

Among others concerned about the fate of government-sponsored medical research after the war was Mrs. Albert D. Lasker. She didn't know quite what to do about the matter, but she was determined to see that if the existing machinery for research sponsorship were dismantled, the fiscal momentum would nonetheless be preserved.[1]

Mary Lasker had long been interested in medical science, and in 1942 she persuaded her husband to join her in establishing a foundation to support medical research. They put up $50,000 to do so and determined to use the income from that investment in such a way as to attract more money and more attention to the scientific search for disease cures. The Lasker Foundation shortly commenced an annual series of awards to medical and biological scientists whose research efforts advanced the cause of better health, awards that became as prestigious as any given in the United States.[2] Mrs. Lasker also began an effort to streamline the American Cancer Society and ultimately was able to increase its budget by quantum proportions.

Albert Lasker had himself intermittently been interested in medical research. In the 1930's, having already made a small fortune as a pioneer in modern advertising, he gave $1 million to the University of Chicago to establish a medical research institute. But he subsequently lost interest in the effort when no visible progress was made on disease cures. In any event, it was Mary who took the lead, though she was usually able to get Albert to join her when her endeavors began to look promising.[3]

Mrs. Lasker brought to the medical research cause a deep emotional commitment. In 1944, when she entered the government policy arena after several years of working with voluntary organizations, she had not yet fully developed those skills in problem analysis, political persuasion, and public opinion molding—of comprehensive, purposeful strategy building—which would later bring her success, envy, and a few foes. At that early point, she brought, first of all, a residual resentment of her own childhood illnesses and of the suffering she had witnessed in family and friends (both her parents died of stroke, and her long-time maid died of cancer) while doctors stood by not knowing what to do. Hers was not just a narrow personal motivation, however; she knew that the National Health Survey of 1936 had shown the state of health of the American people to be poor, and that the draft rejection statistics in the first years of mobilization had dramatized that condition. Mrs. Lasker's own experience with private health-oriented organizations had convinced her that the private sector, alone, could never make sufficient headway against disease. Along with her own personal experience and concern, and the general facts, Mrs. Lasker was endowed with an ability to think in large terms and a simple conviction that something could be done.

She also brought with her to the new phase of her cause—getting government involved in medical research in a big way—an equally remarkable, purposeful friend, Mrs. Daniel Mahoney. Florence Mahoney, who had taken premedical courses in college and who would have become a doctor, she says, had not social and professional pressures got in the way, had had some experience with the political aspects of health. She had tried, not unsuccessfully, to establish mental health programs in Georgia in the late 1930's and had lobbied in that state for birth control. She also had the advantage that her husband (whose late first wife was the daughter of former Governor James Cox of Ohio) owned an interest in the Cox newspaper chain. Hence not only the *Miami Daily News* (of which Mahoney was publisher), but the *Atlanta Journal* and the Dayton and Springfield, Ohio, newspapers could be counted upon to highlight health-related stories, give prominent attention to public opinion polls showing support for health programs, and perhaps most important, support candidates for public office whose platforms the Mahoneys approved of.

Both the Laskers and the Mahoneys knew Senator Claude Pepper of Florida, who in the spring of 1944 was running for re-election. He was also, at that time, planning hearings on the condition of the nation's health. Prompted in part by the health problems and medical successes dramatized by the war years, and in part by the same interest in postwar arrangements and programs that motivated those in the executive branch to take similar looks into the future, Senator Pepper planned the hearings as a general survey. As to where they might lead in policy or program terms, he had an open mind.

When the Laskers visited the Mahoneys in Miami Beach that spring, two decisions were made. Mr. Lasker and Mr. Mahoney would actively support Senator Pepper in his re-election bid, Lasker with money and Mahoney with editorial endorsement. Mrs. Lasker and Mrs. Mahoney would ask Senator Pepper to give particular attention, in the course of his hearings, to the future of medical research. Pepper was, naturally, gratified by the first decision and amenable to the second. That summer he sent two staff members of his Subcommittee on Wartime Health and Education to New York to discuss the research segment of the planned hearings. In reviewing the state of medical research in the country, the Laskers emphasized dollar expenditures (since 1941 over $10 million had been spent on research related to military medicine, while $2 million had been spent, through the Public Health Service, on all other diseases) and illogical priorities. The bulk of PHS research funds were going to health problems, such as rickets, other than those causing the highest percentage of deaths and greatest physical and financial disablement. The Laskers stated their conviction that big-time federal involvement in medical research was essential and offered to help line up witnesses for the hearings.

Because ours has been a research-conscious, even research-oriented society since World War II, it is easy to forget that before Pearl Harbor research was not in a position of high visibility or universally accepted value in our country. In the universities, soon to house great laboratories often involving large teams of scientists, research before the war was but a fractional part of normal campus activity. It was an activity usually small and personal, often disjointed and sometimes, by some academicians, disdained.

If there was a research establishment—comprised of professional laboratory scientists and the foundations and institutes that supported them—it was by and large one which was perfectly content with the prewar style and pace. Federal officials, if asked about the need for change or additional mechanisms or increased authority, usually indicated satisfaction with the status quo, although they sometimes said they could use a little more money to do more of what they were already doing.

Among the public, research, especially medical research, had enjoyed occasional popularity. By the time the proposed cancer research act was scheduled for hearings in 1937 a drumfire of support was being heard in the capital from all corners of the country. Newspapers editorialized in favor of the bill; local organizations adopted supporting resolutions; thousands of letters and telegrams poured in upon the people's representatives in Congress. This focused expression of national sentiment brought government action. Such bursts of popular enthusiasm are not sustained for long, however. The Cancer Institute was established and quietly began its work, which quickly receded from popular attention.

The lack of deep, widespread commitment to medical research as a means of improving the health of the nation, before the war, is perhaps best illustrated by the fact that the American Society for the Control of Cancer spent its efforts and funds on every aspect of the dread disease except research into its causes. Indeed, it was the Laskers' experience with that organization that produced two convictions which, added to their already established commitment to research, motivated them to try to move government in the desired direction after the war.

During the first weeks of the year 1945, Mary Lasker and a newly enlisted ally, Emerson Foote (one of Albert's young business partners, to whom he had given part of his corporation when he retired in 1942), began a special fund-raising effort for the American Society for the Control of Cancer. It was "special" in a very concrete way: the Society had agreed to their conditions that at least one-quarter of the funds thus raised would be spent on research, and that the board of directors of the Society would be changed to include at least fifty percent laymen—both radical innovations for the organization. In only a couple of months, Mrs. Lasker and Mr. Foote had raised over a hundred thousand dollars, most of it generated out of an article in *Readers' Digest* for which they had arranged. The first money, at their insistence, was used to hire a fund-raising staff. Impressed at his wife's early success, Albert Lasker joined the effort and helped to get others involved, including Elmer Bobst of the drug firm of Hoffman, LaRoche, James S. Adams of Standard Brands, and Eric Johnston of the motion picture industry. Using all the skills and techniques of Madison Avenue, and drawing in as many friends as possible, this small group raised $4 million for the cancer society in 1945, in contrast with the $780,000 that had been raised the previous year. (Mr. and Mrs. Mahoney chaired the Miami area effort and raised the local giving from less than $1,000 to $55,000.) In 1946 the Lasker group raised $10 million, and the new board of directors, with Lasker now a member, changed the name of the organization to the American Cancer Society.

The convictions that crystallized from that experience were, first, that when the potential benefits of medical research were dramatized, the American people would support the effort to a far greater degree than had ever been realized; but second, that even the greatly larger amounts of private money that could be raised would not be sufficient to make maximum headway against those diseases that claimed thousands of lives each year. The federal government must become a major continuing participant in the cause.

Some disagreed. Dr. Frank B. Jewett, president of the National Academy of Sciences and head of Bell Telephone Laboratories, one of the four men President Roosevelt had called in to help develop and direct the wartime research effort, thought the government research enterprise should be scaled down after the war ended. Taking an elitist view, Jewett argued that "a large infusion of funds would dilute the quality of American science." [4] Besides, he said, philanthropy and industry, could meet the need: "The amounts of money involved in support of first-class fundamental science research—the only kind that is worthwhile—are infinitesimally small in comparison with national income. The values of this kind of research are measured in terms of men's minds, not in quantities of money." [5]

Albert Lasker's experience, by contrast, led him to believe that money was always an efficacious agent in putting men's minds to work on a problem; and where some money did not turn the trick, more money probably would.

In any case, the medical research environment, when the Lasker-Mahoney combine began its operations in 1944, was one in which most laboratory researchers and their sponsors were satisfied with the pace of progress; those directing wartime research activities were divided on the need for continuing large-scale, special federal programs; private agencies were concentrating on care and prevention but not on cure through research; and members of Congress evidenced only occasional concern, generally coinciding with periodic outbursts of popular enthusiasm, and evidenced ambivalence if not confusion in the face of various research policy approaches being advanced.

That Senator Pepper was willing to focus special attention on the problem of medical research was, in the judgment of the Laskers and their friends, an important step forward. And there were other good signs. At the National Conference on the Problems of Medical Care in 1944, Dr. Alan Gregg of the Rockefeller Foundation "called attention to the contrast with procedures in industrial studies, in which corporations made funds available for work planned over long periods." [6] Reacting to Gregg's statement, the *New York Times* asked editorially why a national medical foundation

> should not plan long-run programs in the same manner . . . Caring minds have never had more than half a chance to demonstrate what medical research can really accomplish . . . It is little short of a disgrace that virtually nothing is known about arthritis, that the conquest of cancer is still far off . . . If we had only the haphazard grant-in-aid system, the chances are that we would not yet have electron tubes . . . and television would still only be a dream. No industrial laboratory would think of conducting research as it is now conducted in medicine. [7]

When Pepper's hearings on postwar medical research got under way in December 1944, the committee heard from 16 witnesses, half of them from the federal government. [8] At least half the others were called at the suggestion of Mrs. Lasker and her friends and included Dr. Cornelius P. Rhoads, on leave as director of Memorial Hospital to head the Army's Chemical Warfare Medical Division. Three or four witnesses are not many; but if all of them are successful doctors and scientists who agree on the need for continuing federal aid for medical research after the war, and call for big money for any such program, the impact is significant. It was, especially in view of the reluctance of some of the government representatives to stake out such clear positions.

Dr. Henry S. Sims of Columbia's College of Physicians and Surgeons, citing statistics that were compiled (he reported) by Mrs. Albert D. Lasker, told chairman Pepper that there was "unanimous agreement that the present sources of peace-time medical research are woefully inadequate." He wanted to see the country move from the less than $5 million spent (by private foundations) in 1940 to $10 million in 1945, twice the amount shortly to be recommended by Dr. Bush. Dr. Sims continued: "And if this amount were increased progressively until $50,000,000 is available in 1953 and each year thereafter, I believe this could be profitably spent for important research on urgent medical problems." Further, Dr. Sims made a recommendation that fell right in line with the Lasker approach: "Any new source of support should be distributed equitably, according to the importance of the medical problems . . . If the federal government is to support peacetime research, I recommend . . . the distributing agency apportion the money according to the number of yearly deaths in the United States from these diseases or groups of diseases or the disabling conditions produced." [9]

Claude Pepper was convinced. Concluding his hearings, he was willing to wait for the Bush report before proceeding to "formulate a program by which the Federal Government can really be helpful." Meanwhile, on the fundamental principal, he agreed with Albert and Mary Lasker and Florence Mahoney: "The volume of research which is carried out in the medical field should, in my opinion, not be limited by lack of money." [10] The next question was which mechanism to choose.

Mrs. Lasker also wanted to be sure the President had not overlooked the issue of postwar medical research. Through her friend Anna Rosenberg, she transmitted a memo to Roosevelt in the fall of 1944 urging that civilian medical problems not be lost sight of as wartime research programs were disestablished.

Vannevar Bush was already considering a research conversion plan in which science could be supported by government in a less fettered way than he thought Senator Kilgore's proposal provided. He shortly composed a draft of a letter from

President Roosevelt to himself asking for recommendations on four major points: how to share U.S. scientific knowledge with the rest of the world, given the need to protect our security; how to wage "the war of science against disease"; what the government could do to aid research efforts of public and private organizations; and how the U.S. could best develop good scientific talent in adequate numbers. The precise impact of Mrs. Lasker's memorandum on this draft is unclear,[11] but the letter to Bush which the President signed on November 17, 1944, stated a premise (for asking how the government should go about waging war on disease) which came to be recognized as a central Lasker theme: "The fact that the annual deaths in this country from one or two diseases alone are far in excess of the total number of lives lost by us in battle during this war alone should make us conscious of the duty we owe future generations." [12]

It took five years for the National Science Foundation legislation to pass Congress in a form acceptable to President Truman.[13] And it took Mrs. Mahoney and Mrs. Lasker four years to conclude that the Public Health Service might provide a suitable vehicle for carrying the nation into a new era of medical research.

Initially they were not impressed with the possibility that an existing agency, the Public Health Service—National Institute of Health, might perform the desired role, despite Dr. Dyer's calling special attention to that alternative in his appearance before the Pepper subcommittee. If they had been intrigued by the knowledge that statutory authority to do the job was already on the books, they were not yet convinced that the leaders of NIH were the men of vision needed to accomplish it. They were bothered by Dr. Dyer's statement that NIH had never had its budget request denied by the Bureau of the Budget or the Appropriations Committees of Congress.[14] No wonder, they thought—those budgets had been of such inconsequential amounts.

Between the time Mrs. Mahoney and she got Senator Pepper to focus his attention on The Cause in 1944 and her ultimate decision in 1948, Mrs. Lasker first bet on a National Medical Research Foundation which Senator Pepper was planning to propose. Then, when Pepper decided in the spring of 1945 that his plan could be incorporated into a revised Kilgore bill, Mrs. Lasker gave up on the separate foundation and subsequently supported a committee of scientists who were campaigning for the Magnuson bill.

Matthew Neely, back in Congress on the House side after four years as Governor of West Virginia, provided one diversion in the interim. In 1946 he introduced a new version of his old cancer bill, with Claude Pepper sponsoring the measure in the Senate. This time Neely wanted the federal government to put up $100 million, to be spent as best and promisingly as possible (for, among other things, the convocation of a panel of world experts) and to remain on tap until expended.[15] Mr. and Mrs. Lasker supported the measure until the wording was changed, on the Senate side, placing the proposed funds under the jurisdiction of the Surgeon General. At that point Mr. Lasker, who had gotten the American Cancer Society to support rather than oppose the Neely bill, withdrew his support, having decided after a conversation with the Surgeon General that Public Health Service officials were not sufficiently interested in or imaginative about research. Mrs. Lasker had found at least one PHS officer, Leonard Scheele, who had given her greater confidence in the agency as a research sponsor.

If Mrs. Lasker was not utterly relentless in pursuing the creation of a medical research foundation in the several years after the war ended, one reason was that she was working on other related matters. She had, for example, with her husband, long tried to convince her friends who were close to the President that an essential feature of any meaningful health program for the country would be a system of national health insurance. President Truman presented to Congress, in September 1945, the first presidential message on health (which his predecessor had agreed to do), with its controversial proposal for a national insurance plan to be underwritten by the government. Mrs. Lasker had urged the President to submit such a message; and Judge Samuel Rosenman implied the Laskers' important involvement in the President's decision by asking them to form a committee to elicit support for the four-point health plan, and to take out advertisements in some of the country's largest newspapers announcing such support. They complied, and the Committee on the Nation's Health was created. Agreeing to support the effort and serve on the Committee were, among others, Mrs. Franklin D. Roosevelt, Gardner Cowles, Henry Kaiser, Mr. and Mrs. Mahoney, and Governor Cox.

It may be questioned whether a buoyant, prosperous, and unthreatened nation can ever be galvanized into action on any front. The urgency of the depression and the imminence of war each brought national unity enabling bold decisions and forward action, spawning national policies and programs to implement them, in a way and at a pace remarkably different from the usual indirect and incremental approach to lesser national needs, smaller public problems.

Great immediate crises often produce strong, swift consensus. Other needs or problems, however central or pervasive, mainly seem to whet personal intellectual appetites and prolong uncompromising positions; seem to insure prompt inaction and, ultimately, if compromise fails, to produce only partial, piecemeal response.

What gives rise to amazement is not that, in contrast to speedy decisions about national research policy when the war began, it took five years from the war's end to hammer out a plan for having the government continue its support of general science. Rather, what puzzles is simply that broad, solid experience seems not to have triumphed over preconceived, personal fears. At the end of the war, many scientists whose total personal and professional sustenance had been provided by government suddenly again distrusted government; and many important public officials whose success in attaining the great objective had been incalculably aided by scientists now indicated reciprocal distrust. The crisis experience had not only illuminated the larger problem but it had also suggested the possibility of an answer. Yet the answer that had worked so well in the crisis was the first one dismissed by the solution seekers.

Dr. Richards tried to explain the contrasting attitudes of medical scientists in war and peace:

> War itself defines the medical problems which must be attacked . . . Peacetime research . . . must be directed at nothing less than the physical and mental advancement of the whole Nation.
>
> It must also be realized that the groundwork of an accelerated approach to solutions of these war problems had already been prepared by the unhurried work of a host of investigators during past decades, many of them working on problems which they regarded as fundamental and from which they may have had little anticipation of practically useful application. These same investigators, stimulated by war necessities and ardently eager to make their capacities useful to the fighting men, changed not only the tempo of their work but also their points of view. Focusing on the practical usefulness of past discoveries and those to come, they have pooled their knowledge and experience, ideas and efforts, and from such pools have come the advances which the low mortality statistics from the fighting fronts are now revealing.
>
> The question arises with what stimulus to replace in the hearts of investigators the ardor for service to the Nation which imminent national danger has provided. And can a Government control, so understanding and so flexible, be created that the imaginations and the scientific passions of the investigators will not be inhibited? [16]

Not many persons at that point were absolutely sure of how to accomplish the task. Some believed that money would be a sufficient stimulus. Few scientists would have admitted that possibility, and those administering science research funds and dealing with scientists every day couldn't have admitted it even if they believed it. The problem, Dr. Dyer told Senator Pepper in 1944, was not one of money for cancer research but of finding good men who were already interested and trained. On the other hand, some scientists agreed that the availability of money could be a deciding factor in choosing among research fields.[17] Dr. Leonard Scheele, former director of the National Cancer Institute and Surgeon General, recalls that when the Cancer Institute was created in 1937 his mentor in the Public Health Service, Dr. Joe Mountain (a specialist in public health methods), suggested that he take advantage of both the purely scientific and the professional career possibilities that would be available in the Institute because of its grand appropriation.[18] Still, the question was on the mechanism; for that, plus financial commitment and stated goals, would constitute actual policy.

While the debate on that key issue droned on, side issues arose. In 1945 Congressman Percy Priest (D., Tenn.) of the Interstate and Foreign Commerce Committee introduced a bill which he felt would help meet another need pointed up by the draft statistics of the war years: mental health problems. The measure would establish a mental health division within the Public Health Service and, among other things, provide funds for the training of psychiatrists, in shorter supply throughout the country than was the case for any other branch of medicine. Mrs. Lasker and Mrs. Mahoney approved of the idea, and after consultations with Priest, whom they had not known before, went to see their old friend Senator Pepper. Pepper then introduced the measure in the Senate.

Mrs. Lasker's multiple health legislation interests and her husband's poor health, which necessitated frequent travel to Florida and California, posed problems for Mrs. Lasker. She was working on the $100 million cancer research bill in the Congress, trying to help develop national support for the health insurance plan, and attempting to settle in her own mind and in conversation with colleagues the question of how best to arrange a medical research support system, when the Priest bill came up. Other good ideas and promising proposals had failed, she recognized, simply because there was no one to push them through the inevitable tangles of the legislative maze. Why not, she suggested to the National Committee for Mental Hygiene, employ a lobbyist to follow the measure, coordinate support for it, and keep key supporters in and out of Congress advised of progress and problems? The Committee was amenable—if Mrs. Lasker would put up the money. She did, and Mr. Lynn Adams was hired. Within approximately one year after its introduction, the National Mental Health Act was signed by the President on July 4, 1946.[19]

As in the case of the Cancer Act nine years earlier, a number of factors combined to produce this landmark legislation. The Public Health Service itself was interested in expanding its role in the mental health field. At least, it permitted the director of its Mental Hygiene Division, Dr. Robert Felix, to present his plan for a system of community mental health programs to Oscar Ewing, head of the Federal Security Agency, in 1944. With Ewing's approval, Felix and his colleague Mary Switzer went to see a Congressman they thought would be sympathetic, Percy Priest. When Priest arranged hearings before his subcommittee of the Interstate and Foreign Commerce Committee, he and the two other members present that day—Congressmen Clarence Brown (R., Ohio) and Charles Wolverton (R., N.J.), the latter chairman of the full committee—heard testimony from Felix and from representatives of the National Committee on Hygiene. But they also heard a surprise witness.

A young man in Marine uniform stood up in the audience and asked the chairman if he could be permitted to address the committee. Priest consented. The Marine told a brief story of his war experience, of ordeals that caused mental breakdown, and of the availability of professional help and treatment facilities so rare that he was being treated at St. Elizabeth's Hospital. Dr. Felix remembers his plea to the committee: "For God's sake, help us. Do something. Give us a chance." The Congressmen could not have been unmoved.[20]

As the bill moved along, Mrs. Mahoney got the Cox papers to feature stories about it; the *Miami Daily News'* endorsement was particularly pleasing to Senator Pepper, its Senate sponsor. Eugene Myer was also interested in the bill, and the *Washington Post,* which he published, gave it full supportive treatment. The bill had friends in Congress (Senators Taft, Aiken, LaFollete, Vandenberg, and Hill were co-sponsors), in the affected agency, among interest groups, and in the press. Yet such support was not nearly so pervasive as that for the Cancer Act of 1937. The new element which seemed to fill the gap between massive, intense pressure and congressional action was a full-time, single-minded, paid lobbyist. This was a lesson Mrs. Lasker and her friends took seriously.

There was one other lesson she and Mrs. Mahoney learned. Pleased with their first completed success—as they thought of it—they congratulated themselves and began working on other projects. Then someone asked them how much money had actually been appropriated to begin work. They answered that $17 million had been authorized. Yes, was the reply, but how much did the Congress appropriate for the coming year? Puzzled, they asked what the difference was between authorization and appropriation. They did not forget the answer.

In November 1944 the Surgeon General of the Public Health Service, Dr. Thomas Parran, proposed a six-point health program for the nation after the war. The goals were: 1) a sanitary environment, 2) an adequate hospital system, 3) an expanded public health service, 4) augmented research in health, 5) medical personnel in adequate numbers, and 6) a national medical care program. It was, minus "sanitary environment" and "expanded public health service," a harbinger of the presidential program a year later. On the research side, Parran wanted to see "enough research to reduce the enormous toll of mental disease, cancer, heart disease, arthritis, and to suppress plagues of typhus and tropical diseases, and to conquer dental caries." [21]

Despite Parran's outline, and perhaps because of more immediate organizational goals—gearing up to be able to handle the transfer of wartime research contracts and, before that, securing the necessary legislative authorization—little progress actually seemed to be in the making on those programmatic goals affecting, or at least relating to, the people directly. There are evidences of real foresight on the part of some top Public Health Service officials, including Dr. Parran, during the late years of the war. But even if they had good, long-range ideas, they were not going to enjoy that favorite bureaucratic luxury of setting their own pace.

Peace brought with it such rapid dissolution of consensus on goals that large policy decisions were ineluctably postponed. It also freed up Congressmen and special interest groups to begin, once more, pushing their own special notions and programs; to begin vying once more for national attention (or at the very least local prominence) on grounds of having the most original, beneficent proposals, sure to bring greatest good to the American people if only the Congress and the bureaucracy could be persuaded to accept them. Cancer was still a favorite theme; thus the revival of Senator Neely's theme of just putting up enough money and getting the job done.

The Public Health Service was, in those years, in the difficult position of having to demonstrate authority, experience, capacity, and vision, so that it would not be overlooked as a possible repository for the new, large-scale medical research funds which a combination of forces were inevitably going to produce; and, on the other hand, of having to be certain that it did not accept greater responsibilities, or greater sums of money, than it could effectively cope with. It was a tightrope that NIH particularly was going to become quite accustomed to walking over the years.

No, Dr. Dyer responded to "Governor" Neely of the House Appropriations Subcommittee in the spring of 1946, NIH could not use any extra money for cancer studies. The $1.75 million requested was all that could be soundly used.[22] The Public Health Service "5-Year Plan" called for an annual expenditure of approximately $1.5 million, and the NIH leadership wanted to stay with that figure.[23] Neely charged that "the cancer people have adopted a defeatist attitude." [24]

That incident caused the stir that led the Lasker lobby to fight for the Neely Cancer Bill providing additional millions of dollars to be expended by a new agency outside the jurisdiction of the Surgeon General. Dr. Parran sought to explain to the House committee holding hearings on the bill that his colleague, Dr. Dyer, had only meant that NIH was restricted in the amount of money they could effectively use by available researchers, and that at that moment they didn't know whether additional researchers would be available to join in the fight to conquer cancer.[25] That explanation being not good enough, and not just the millions of dollars but control over a new cancer effort about to slip away from them, the Public Health Service authorized Dr. Leonard Scheele, associate director of the National Cancer Institute, to present a further explanation, a slightly different approach. He told Congress that while the Institute probably could not use all of the proffered additional dollars the very next year, NIH had decided that it would nonetheless be a good thing if the Congress were to authorize a higher appropriations ceiling, so that as soon as the Cancer Institute built up its capacity to effectively use the extra money it could proceed to do so. Neely was apparently satisfied; and so was the bill's Senate sponsor, Senator Pepper, who agreed to rewrite it so as to provide the new money to the Public Health Service rather than to a new agency.[26]

It was more because the session was by then getting "late"—July was considered late in those days—than that Albert Lasker withdrew from the measure his support and that of the Cancer Society (Mary Lasker's continued) that the Senate objected to taking up the bill by special request. But the fact that both a Senate and a House committee had favored such an increase in cancer research funds, and had not been sure such funds ought to be encharged to the National Institute of Health, gave Dr. Parran, Dr. Dyer, and their colleagues something new to ponder. The next year, the National Institute of Health asked the Congress for "big money"; its budget went from less than $8 million in fiscal 1947 to over $26 million in fiscal 1948. The cost of carrying out wartime contracts was one reason for the big increase, but another factor was that the top bureaucrats decided they must get ahead to stay alive. Under Dr. Scheele the National Cancer Institute asked for, instead of a mere increment over its 1947 budget of $1.8 million, over $14 million. The Institute would do its best, the message to Congress and the emerging lobbyists said, to help conquer cancer.

To take a further look at science policy needs, and to create new momentum for decisions that still needed to be made, President Truman in October 1946 asked his President's Scientific Research Board "to investigate and report on the entire scientific program of the federal government." The Board's report, referred to by the name of its chairman, John Steelman, was presented to the President one year later. It posited a strong conviction of the nation's interest in medical research: "The conquest of disease, like the conquest of hunger, is of primary concern to the people. The conquest of time, space, power and substitutes for natural resources—even for peaceful purposes—is secondary, for without a healthy population, those would be empty victories to the nation." How could the conquest of disease be achieved? "Two major steps are needed promptly to assist in overcoming those barriers to realizing recent gains in medical science and further progress. They are: Provision of substantial additional funds for training and research at the earliest possible moment; formulation of a national policy on medical research." [27]

Lest those recommendations seem so obvious and so vague as to be innocuous, the report specifically recommended a gradual increase in medical research funds to attain an annual expenditure of $300 million by 1957; and it suggested that the national policy and a comprehensive program to fulfill it should be designed by a new medical research committee.

The Hoover Commission was in the process of trying to do that (among other things), but when its final recommendation emerged, urging the establishment of a national medical administration with PHS and its research division as one component, some of the most distinguished Commission members —Dean Acheson, Senator George Aiken, James Rowe—dissented.[28] Would the issue—of national science policy, including national medical research policy—ever get settled?

Policy, Daniel Greenberg suggests, "is essentially an ordering of priorities." [29] To accept that definition is to accept the possibility that policy can be made according to a logical, synoptic process necessitating explicit agreements and goals; or, that policy can evolve out of a series of marginal moves and uncoordinated decisions, permitted by vague agreement on broad goals but not necessitating specific accords or ordered sequences of action. Policy, that is, can evolve de facto out of an aggregate of decisions and commitments only indirectly related to one another. If nothing else was clear about the national medical research policy in the later 1940's, one thing was: it was not going to be established by hard consensus on a grand design. It would be fragmentary and incremental; in short, evolutionary.

Because the Public Health Service seemed only to be able to react—sometimes reluctantly, always slowly—to priorities urged by others, it was a vulnerable agency in that govern-mental *bouleversement* of the immediate postwar years. Its leaders had ideas of their own, but somehow the image it pro-jected was one of little movement despite occasional thought-fulness. Dr. Parran had spoken of the need to tackle the prob-lem of heart disease in 1944; Dr. Norman Topping, whom Parran relied on for postwar planning and priority-setting on various occasions, had inserted into the Steelman Report of 1947 specific mention of heart disease as a high priority item among research needs. But little occurred to demonstrate that the National Institute of Health was going to meet needs it claimed to recognize, until Mary Lasker moved on that subject.

Mrs. Lasker had first favored an approach to conquering heart disease similar to that advanced most recently by Matthew Neely for cancer: set aside $100 million to remain available until spent for every imaginative approach to the problem that could be developed by the world's leading experts. Early in 1947, she mailed a copy of a draft bill to her loyal friend Senator Pepper, who introduced such a measure a week later, on February 16.

There was one new problem, however. The Republican vic-tory in the congressional elections of 1946 had denied Pepper his committee chairmanship. He could no longer singlehandedly accomplish missions suggested by Mrs. Lasker. There was, he told her, one possibility that ought to be explored. Senator Styles Bridges of New Hampshire, now chairman of the Ap-propriations Committee, had not been unsympathetic to medical research in the past; besides, he had recently had a heart attack. Perhaps he would be interested to know that no funds had ever been earmarked for research into heart disease and other circu-latory ailments by the National Institute of Health.

Senator Bridges was interested, and even offered to hold hearings on a deficiency appropriation for NIH so as to provide immediate funds for heart research if Mrs. Lasker could help line up appropriate witnesses. Such a hearing was arranged in late May. Mrs. Lasker listened with pleasure as representatives of the American Heart Association told Senator Bridges of the need for earmarked funds. She listened with even greater pleasure as Senator Bridges expressed agreement with these experts and said that such funds would be provided. Whether Senator Bridges knew it or not, Mrs. Lasker had mentally earmarked funds for his next campaign, coming up the following year.

Dr. Leonard Scheele, whose strategy in 1946 had helped save the Cancer Institute from the ire of Congress and even from the competition of a rival agency, and who became director of the NCI the next year, was chosen by President Truman as Surgeon General in April 1948 to succeed Dr. Parran. Florence Mahoney and Mary Lasker thought it was a particularly good choice, for Scheele had demonstrated a flexibility and a vision they liked.

In turn, Scheele thought it might be enormously valuable for the National Institute to have friends like Mrs. Lasker and Mrs. Mahoney, whose contacts with the White House were solid and whose friends in Congress could probably help insure that NIH would become the single most important instrument in any national medical research program. Dr. Parran had had occasional contact with the new lobbyists, but Dr. Scheele was accessible to them any time.

With new friends in important positions, the Lasker-Mahoney team became more relaxed and more direct and, finally, more amenable to seeing NIH become *the* national medical research foundation. Shortly before he became Surgeon General, Scheele received a telephone call from Mary Lasker. The Congress had recently demonstrated its interest in seeing heart research stepped up, she said, and the NIH keeps saying it's interested. Why not establish a heart institute similar to the Cancer Institute so as to dramatize that interest and make it possible to get more support to do bigger things? Scheele thought it was a good idea but suggested Mrs. Lasker talk with Surgeon General Parran about it. When Parran made no objection, Scheele drafted legislation patterned closely after the Cancer Act: it provided for the conduct of heart research within the proposed institute, for grants to outside institutions; and for training grants in science and clinical medicine. It contained two new features, one of which was particularly gratifying to universities (grant funds for research facility construction) and the other especially pleasing to Mrs. Lasker (the allowance for laymen to serve on the advisory councils). Since this was to be the second "categorical research" institute, NIH would now become the National Institutes of Health.

The bill was introduced in the Senate by Senator Bridges and co-sponsored by Senators Ives (R., N.Y.), Murray (D., Mont.), and Pepper. Once again the Congress moved quickly, as it had done a decade earlier in creating the Cancer Institute. In a remarkably short time the Senate and the House enacted the measure designed, its sponsors said, to conquer what had become the nation's number one killer, heart disease. On June 16, 1948, President Truman signed the measure into law;[30] straightway, Surgeon General Scheele appointed Mrs. Lasker as the first layman to serve on a medical research advisory council.

The medical research lobby was firmly ensconced, and its alliance with the National Institutes of Health had begun. NIH would probably be *the* national medical research foundation, regardless of what finally happened to the National Science Foundation proposal. Attacks would be made on specific diseases. More money would be sought, and obtained. National policy on medical research—with goals, implementary machinery, funds, and fighting friends—was beginning to crystallize.

That fall Mary and Albert Lasker made a contribution to Styles Bridges' campaign. Having been assistant treasurer of the Republican National Committee in earlier years, Albert Lasker naturally tended to favor Republican candidates with his campaign contributions. But he often made them whimsically, sending a check to a candidate whom he hardly knew because he had formed a favorable impression of him on indirect evidence. Mary persuaded him to be a little more systematic and purposeful in his campaign giving: Bridges deserved their support not because he was a Republican or simply a "good man" but because he had helped advance a cause they were interested in. Bridges had proven to be a friend, and proven friends deserved proven friends. "The Laskers," an acquaintance later said, "don't buy votes, they reward votes." And though the Laskers' contributions were usually modest, their willingness to show appreciation in this way provided encouragement to those members of Congress whose interest in the cause of medical research was less than passionate. Typically, as Albert saw Mary's approach begin to succeed, he adopted it as his own. He said to a friend: "I can spend a few thousands of dollars and produce millions of dollars for health."

IV Federal Aid for Medical Education:
The AMA and Avenues Blocked

One cause for which Albert Lasker could not spend seed money
and produce the flowering of a program was that of a national
health insurance system, the linch-pin in President Truman's
five-point health program for the nation. The Laskers' Committee for the Nation's Health was utterly unsuccessful on that
front, for there it met formidable opposition. Not simply opposition of a few key figures in key positions, the kind of opposition that can be gotten around if it cannot be brought around.
This was organized, professional, well-heeled opposition claiming a wide popular base. It was the opposition of the American
Medical Association, and the campaign it mounted made the
Laskers' campaign seem puny indeed.

The origins of the proposed national health insurance plan
and the bitter struggle over it, lasting thirty years and reaching
particularly bloody proportions politically in the late 1940's
and again in the early 1960's, have been recorded in detail elsewhere. Richard Harris, among others, has told of how the AMA
raised a multimillion-dollar war chest and spent most of that
with a public relations agency to beat this and any other program it considered "socialized medicine." [1] Indeed, the political
power of the American Medical Association was commonly
recognized and uncommonly real. The implications of its war
against national health insurance are important for the present
story simply because they suggest how fortunate it was for the
cause of medical research that *that* particular governmental
enterprise was not singled out for attack.

What is not so well known, and what underscores the importance of the AMA's neutrality on medical research—a neutrality that became permanently fixed during its wars against

other programs—is how the organization killed an early post-war proposal to provide direct federal aid to medical schools and medical students, another idea contained in President Truman's plan and subsequently refined and strengthened by the Congress.

Although he urged federal government support for medical education, President Truman apparently did not hold to the particular fear that became the basis of a consensus almost producing congressional action: fear that the country would soon be faced with a severe shortage of physicians. Emphasizing that the problem was one of the right number of doctors not being in the right places, the President thought the total supply was adequate.[2]

Others doubted that. In May 1945 the secretary of the American Medical Association's Council on Medical Education told the Senate Military Affairs Committee that existing institutional capacities and class sizes would produce one-half of the predicted need for 35,000 more physicians by 1948.[3] A little over two years later, in October 1947, the new secretary of the same AMA Council expressed somewhat less concern, contending that "the maximum deficit that could possibly be forecast for 1960 does not exceed 15,000 physicians." [4]

Almost every study, and every student, of the subject for the next several years supported the belief of the developing shortage of physicians. They were unanimous on the other reason for federal aid: financial crisis among medical schools all over the country. In one of his few public appearances in behalf of causes in which he believed and for which he worked so skillfully behind the scenes, Albert Lasker testified before the House Interstate and Foreign Commerce Committee in May 1949 on the proposed comprehensive "National Health Plan," and gave his impression of the need.

> I have gotten into contact and had lengthy exchange of views with the heads of the greatest medical schools in the

United States and I know directly from them that they are on the verge of a financial catastrophe. I do not believe— and I may be mistaken—I may be speaking in too lurid terms—that there is a medical school in the country which, unless large private funds and Government funds, both, are made available, and I am for the raising of both—can in 5 years fail to have a crisis.[5]

Dr. Alan Gregg, director of Medical Sciences for the Rockefeller Foundation, said in the spring of 1949: "I wonder if Americans understand how alarming is the future of medical education in this country. Unless our medical schools receive substantially larger sums for their essential expenses, we shall not in the future have care which modern medicine could provide. For it is only through the hands of men and women trained by our medical schools that society provides itself with medical care." [6]

The American Medical Association was becoming increasingly skeptical about any doctor shortage, as its representatives testified before the Senate Labor and Public Welfare Committee in 1949. But the AMA too attested to the critical need for funds for medical schools and accepted the proposition that the federal government, under certain safeguards, could properly assist.[7]

Senator Robert Taft of Ohio ("Mr. Republican") in the same year acknowledged that "it seems to be universally agreed that more personnel is necessary as health service is expanded by whatever means it may be expanded." [8]

In 1949 President Truman's health program for the nation was presented anew. It was as comprehensive a plan as Congress had ever actively considered or would ever consider in one piece again. Sponsored in the Senate by Democrats James Murray, Robert Wagner, Claude Pepper, and others and on the House side by Democrat Andrew Biemiller of Wisconsin, the "National Health Program" not only provided for a prepayment health insurance system (the Wagner-Murray-Dingell proposal which Congress had already seen and would struggle over repeatedly during the coming decades); it also provided for expansion of the Hill-Burton Hospital Construction Act, enacted in 1946, and for expansion of medical research; and its most novel features were proposals for direct aid for medical schools and, as a separate provision, scholarships for medical students.[9]

The American Medical Association had already geared up for war against national health insurance. The proposed intrusion of the federal government into medical education also concerned them mightily; they would have liked to sidetrack that proposal without diverting attention, and the coordinated efforts of their membership, from the principal evil of the moment—the insurance package.

Associates of Senator Murray say that the packaging of health insurance, hospital construction, medical research, and federal aid to medical education in a single bill was a calculated strategy to avoid having the American Medical Association continue in their usual stance of opposition to almost every measure calling for systematic federal involvement in improving the nation's health. Except for "public health" measures (such as tuberculosis and malaria control) and hospital construction, the AMA had feared any federal health program as a Trojan horse. Senator Murray and his colleagues were not so naïve as to think that by putting all the mentioned features in one bill they would overwhelm their persistent and well-organized opposition. They did believe that the AMA would find it difficult to wage total war against all parts of the omnibus bill: because the medical profession was not of as powerful persuasion on the other features as on compulsory health insurance and, in any case, because opposition to the total bill would throw into dramatic relief their total opposition to almost any bill—their persistent, essential negativism.

The proposed National Health Program of 1949 could be held up as a model of sound legislative planning; of an intelligent, thorough, and balanced policy plan. Its premise was that "the health of its people is the foundation of our Nation's strength, productivity and wealth," and its provisions included all the basic ingredients to strengthen that "foundation." [10]

National policy is rarely established on so direct and comprehensive a design. And it was not so established in this instance. The National Health Program of 1949 largely became national policy on a piecemeal basis over the next twenty years. (Indeed, all of it *will* become law if the last provision, national health insurance, is to be enacted sometime in the next several years— perhaps by 1975, the thirtieth anniversary of its introduction in Congress.) But the 1949 plan, as and when it was first proposed, was more a matter of immediate political strategy than of sound, long-range planning; and its Senate sponsors can be congratulated for their success—their one-time, short-term success.

The American Medical Association predictably concentrated their opposition on the health insurance plan. One of their witnesses was Dr. Lowell S. Goin, president of the California Physicians' Service; Goin opposed the bill, he indicated, not simply as a spokesman for the organized medical profession but "as an American because I am persuaded that this type of legislation is one of the final steps on the road to state socialism." [11] His opposition extended to the provision for aid to students, and he and other AMA representatives sought to undercut the widespread conviction that there was fast developing a critical shortage of medical and related personnel. Dr. Louis H. Bauer, charman of AMA's board of trustees and the organization's spokesman at the Senate hearings in March 1947 argued that "since 1940 the population has increased 13 percent and the number of physicians has increased 15 percent.[12] I do not mean to infer that we do not need more doctors; I think we do need more, but I say we are getting them steadily." Besides, he added, "you must remember that illness is diminishing." [13]

The AMA would not oppose extension of the Hill-Burton Act to help pay for construction projects of various kinds, "locally originated, for rural and other areas in which the need can be shown." [14] Their 12-point program did favor "promotion of medical research through a national science foundation with grants to private institutions," provided, of course, that such institutions have "facilities and personnel sufficient to carry on qualified research." [15] And even if they discounted the doctor shortage, because they feared federal aid to medical education, they could not deny the critical financial situation existing in most medical schools in the country. Nor had they any other plan, at that point, for saving the schools from bankruptcy. AMA was "aware that Federal aid to medical education creates definite hazards to the continued freedom and independence of medical schools." But it acknowledged that "with few exceptions . . . the medical schools and their parent universities have expressed the opinion that, unless additional aid is provided, medical education in this country cannot achieve its full development." [16] Thus did the AMA tacitly accept, though only for one brief moment as it turned out, the idea of federal aid to medical education. That small opening was all the bill's original sponsors needed.

The Senate Subcommittee on Health also considered, in May of 1949, Senator Taft's bill, an alternative to the Democrats' National Health Program. Naturally the Taft bill substituted a "voluntary" health insurance provision for the "compulsory" insurance provision of the Democrats. It did provide, however, for federal aid to medical schools by authorizing direct payment to the schools according to the number of present and "new" students and, like the Murray-Pepper bill, authorizing limited funds for medical school construction. It authorized no scholarship funds, and Senator Taft's colleague, Claude Pepper, asked why.

> Sen. Pepper: You do not make provision in your bill for scholarships for students?
> Sen. Taft: No. Yesterday Mr. Kingsley [acting administrator of the Federal Security Administration, who had

testified for the "Administration Bill"] testified there was
no emergency about that . . . You have four or five times
the number of applicants who are able to pay their way
through . . . But, as I say, in the meantime to try to stimulate and help some schools which might go on the rocks
completely, and to encourage them to keep up their enrollment and perhaps increase it somewhat, we have this
additional money. Most of them take the position that they
cannot increase their enrollment without having increased
facilities and that the effort to give schools $1,700 [which
the Democrats' bill would do] for new students is an incentive for them to put on more than they could properly
educate.[17]

Senator Taft also proposed a commission to study the plight
of medical schools and recommend a permanent program to
follow the five-year "emergency program."

The opening provided for those Senators who sought federal
aid for medical education was quickly seized. A special work
group who subsequently drafted a modified medical education
bill for the Senate committee reported on their unusual service:

It appeared from the testimony of witnesses speaking to
both Title I of the Democrats' bill and Title VI [of the
Taft bill] that with relatively little adjustment of details,
the provisions of S.1679 would be acceptable to the educa-
tors in the professions concerned. All witnesses were, therefore, asked if they could hold themselves available during
the following week to discuss with the staff of the Senate
Labor and Public Welfare Committee the changes which
they considered necessary to insure endorsement of the bill
by the organizations which they represented. All agreed.[18]

A new bill was drafted with not just the cognizance but also
the participation of representatives of the American Medical

Association; carrying the endorsement of a number of medical deans, university heads, and educational associations, it was brought to the Senate in September 1949. The bill provided "a 5-year emergency program of grants and scholarships for education" in medicine and related fields, authorized a commission to study the long-range needs of medical schools, and included the usual provisions "taking care of other purposes." Reported with the endorsement of all but one member of the Senate committee, and with Senator Pepper and Senator Taft jointly managing the floor action, the bill passed the Senate on a voice vote, with no opposing votes heard, on September 23, 1949.[19]

On the House side, the Committee on Interstate and Foreign Commerce likewise favorably reported the measure, with Congressmen Andrew Biemiller and Hugh Scott (R., Pa.) jointly sponsoring amendments to further mollify AMA fears and then jointly urging the bill's passage. All foreseeable barriers to enactment were at last removed.

Funny things sometimes happen on the way to the main forum from a congressional committee. Albert Q. Maisel tells what occurred next: "By then, late in the session, it was necessary for the House Rules Committee to speed action on the measure if the whole House was to vote on it without delay. This procedure promised to be routine." But suddenly the situation changed:

> A small group of insurgent members of the nurses' organizations in Georgia and North Carolina, and the owner of a private hospital in the latter state, got the impression that the measure would somehow set up the American Nursing Association as an accrediting body for all nursing schools—and thus force the closing down, for lack of accreditation, of some of the less qualified schools in the Southern States.
>
> On behalf of this group, Representative Robert L. (Muley) Doughton of North Carolina, protested to the

Rules Committee. The sponsors of the Bill offered to amend the measure to overcome the objection. This satisfied Doughton and he withdrew his protest.

But the Biemiller bill had, by then, become "controversial." The Rules Committee, fearful of setting a precedent that would throw a host of other controversial measures on the House floor in the last two weeks of the session, withheld its approval. The bill was held up until Congress could meet again, in 1950.[20]

Instead the bill died, and with it the possibility of direct federal aid to medical education. It was not exactly a natural death. In fact, it had been plotted. And not for fourteen years would the idea be successfully revived.

The American Medical Association perceived that the National Health Program of 1949 was a legislative strategy paralleling the military prescription that division can lead to conquest. Or at least their advertising representatives, Whitaker and Baxter, did. Clem Whitaker warned of "hidden threats" in the "fringe" provision of aid to medical education. "Instead of being confronted with the task of defeating a revolutionary program of Government medicine, embodied in a single proposal, or in companion bills, we are now faced with a series of measures—disarming in language but dangerous in their provisions—some of which must be beaten and some drastically changed or amended." [21]

Whether it is applied on the military or legislative battlefield, there is an obvious corollary or caveat to the ancient rule: once the foe is divided, or diverted, or overextended, the winning thrust must be quick and sure. Otherwise, the opponent regroups and re-establishes a solid position. The AMA did not take long.

In December 1949, following the September Senate passage of the emergency medical education bill, the AMA's House of Delegates adopted a report that said: "The legislation which has been passed by the Senate contains safeguards that should protect the medical schools from unwarranted interference in their affairs by the Federal Government." [22] But two months later, the AMA added this measure to the long list of bills it opposed. The reason, said Board Chairman Louis Bauer, was that "as the bill is presently drawn, we feel it would give the Government a foot in the door—in fact, probably two feet in the door —for Federal control of medical education. There are certain very drastic amendments which will have to be made to that bill before we can approve it." [23]

Such revisions were made. In the spring of 1950, the House sponsors lowered the subsidy maximums to 30 percent, as the AMA had originally proposed, and spelled out in even greater detail the protections against federal intrusion. The AMA counterstrategy was characterized by Congressman Biemiller as a "stalling-twisting-turning-conniving policy of compromise and-then-oppose-the-compromise." [24] It was also a successful policy. The House Interstate and Foreign Commerce Committee refused four times between June and the end of August— each time by one vote—to send to the House the measure which President Truman had called "the most vital health legislation before Congress." [25]

On June 25, 1950, the Korean War broke out. It made vividly clear the existence of a doctor shortage: the military needed more than 1,500 additional physicians immediately and was estimated to need some 5,000 more if the armed forces grew to 3 million men. The impact on civilian health personnel was serious and obvious. Yet even this dramatic happening, which might have been thought to boost the chances as well as highlight the need for federal aid for medical education, did not persuade the opponents. They continued to oppose, now using the war and its costs and the consequent need to economize as another reason for opposing.

Meanwhile, other evidence developed to confirm the need. Dean Joseph C. Hinsey of Cornell Medical School, chairman of the Executive Council of the Association of American Medical Colleges, polled the Association's membership and reported that 47 favored the bill and 16 opposed it.[26] The Surgeon General's Committee on Medical School Grants and Finances found, in December 1950, the financial crisis of medical schools very real: "The present state of unequal equilibrium in which medical schools now exist cannot continue." [27] The National Fund for Medical Education, incorporated under the honorary chairmanship of Herbert Hoover, tried to raise $40 million from private funds for medical schools, but succeeded in raising only a little over $1 million over a two-year period. The Fund concluded: "Certainly there can be no objection to the use of Federal funds in aid of the medical schools in the face of the emergency that exists today." [28] In February 1950 Dr. Howard A. Rusk, chairman of the Selective Service System's National Advisory Committee on mobilization of medical personnel, as well as chairman of the ongoing Health Resources Advisory Committee to the National Security Board, told the Annual Council on Medical Education and Hospitals—sponsored by, among others, the American Medical Association—that the physician deficit would be 22,000 by 1954, and would remain at that level or greater through the decade, unless immediate remedies were initiated.[29]

Seventeen of the 18 professional associations which had supported the emergency medical education bill in 1949, including the Association of American Medical Colleges, American Dental Association, American Hospital Association, American Nurses Association, American Public Health Association, and American Council on Education, supported it still in the spring and summer of 1951 when it was again brought to the floor of the Senate. One organization had changed its stance from tentative support to outright opposition: the American Medical Association.

Scorning the recent congressional precedent, institutional financial trends, and more numerous organizations and their more relevant expertise, the AMA turned against the bill and killed it. The attack was not limited to direct argument, mobilization, and assault, but included equally potent indirect means. The direct assault was led, in the Senate, by Everett Dirksen, who gave full vocal dressing to the AMA's claimed fears of federal control of health and education. Blocking consideration of the "Emergency Professional Health Training Act of 1951" on Calendar Monday, Senator Dirksen said: "I intend to object to this bill. I object to it politically. I object to it congenitally. I object to it socially and in every other way. I think it is an invasion of the educational field. If we spell this out far enough, and it becomes a pattern, it will only be a question of time until the Federal Government will be dominating the educational field." [30]

The direct attack also included the timeworn technique of a massive barrage of telegrams from constituents to Congressmen. Senator Murray exhorted the Senate not to let this tactic work again. Saying that the AMA hierarchy had contacted key physicians around the country—"perhaps your physician or mine" —to bring pressure on the Congress to defeat the bill, Murray pleaded with his colleagues: "Gentlemen, in the names of the tens of thousands of decent doctors in America, doctors such as you know and I know, I resent this shoddy, indefensible sort of action which was taken in their names. I know we will not allow it to influence our consideration of a bill which means so very much to the welfare of this Nation and of its Armed Services." [31]

It was the indirect attack that proved lethal: simply, the conversion of Senator Taft. Taft had probably joined in sponsoring the emergency medical aid bill somewhat reluctantly at first. He doubted the need for additional doctors, arguing that it was quality and not quantity that was needed in medicine. But the plight of the medical schools was as severe in Ohio as elsewhere, and once the formula was worked out, he seemed to take the bill as his own. In seeking return to the Senate in the 1950 elections, he even used the bill as a campaign plank. In March

1951, speaking about the successor bill to that passed earlier, Taft told the Senate: "So far as the last election is concerned, I must say that in nearly every speech I made in Ohio, I advocated passage of this bill; consequently I do not regard my own election, at least, as a repudiation of a bill which I supported in the last Congress." [32]

The import of Taft's remarks at that time indicate that he was still supportive of the measure. He talked about the problems of "the shortage of facilities in which to train students," and the burden on the medical schools caused by the differential in the cost of tuition and the actual cost of training students. He thought the bill "of such importance that it should be brought before the Senate at the earliest possible moment by the majority leader." [33]

The new bill was finally brought before the Senate by the majority leader, Ernest McFarland (D., Ariz.), in October 1951. Its management was entrusted to a freshman Senator, John Pastore of Rhode Island. An unusual move, associates of committee chairman Murray say that this was simply because the bill was expected to sail through the Senate with no problem. It was, after all, almost identical to that passed "unanimously" by the Senate two years earlier; it was treated as having been unanimously accepted and reported by the Labor and Public Welfare Committee. Chairman Murray scorned the AMA's charges that the bill would lead to federal control. "Imagine," he said, "the Senator from Ohio, Mr. Taft, sponsoring a bill through which the federal government would control state and private universities. You can't imagine it, Mr. President—nor can the American people—nor can the individual doctors of America." [34]

One wonders if Senator Murray, no political slouch, could have at least imagined, if he had not already learned, that Senator Taft was going to join ranks with the AMA and turn against the bill. If he had so perceived, he could have saved the bill's floor manager some shock and no little face.

Taft's ultimate opposition was first revealed as the Senate finally moved to debate the matter in October 1951. He opposed amendments to the bill (one offered by Senator Pastore and a similar one by Senators Richard Russell of Georgia and Robert Kerr of Oklahoma, all Democrats,) which would have offered less money to medical schools for sustaining present enrollment levels and more incentive money to schools to increase their class sizes.[35] On this issue, the medical school deans themselves split; as Committee member Hubert H. Humphrey, one of the strongest supporters of the bill and the amendments, explained: "The amendment was not as desired by the northern medical schools which have large medical enrollments . . . [it] was primarily designed for those areas of the country and those schools that do not have a large medical enrollment . . . designed to increase enrollment in smaller colleges and to give some opportunity for expansion of medical facilities." [36]

Senator Taft reported to the Senate that

> Dean Berry, who is Dean of the Harvard Medical School and chairman of the executive committee of the Association of American Medical Schools, says that he personally will not support the bill if it is so amended . . . He is speaking for the Association. They would rather have no aid at all than to have the bill as amended by the Russell-Kerr amendment. That is also the view of the Dean of the Cornell Medical School. I should say that is the view of the best medical educators in the country. Certainly if they do not want the assistance, this is no time to force it upon them.[37]

The controversy, say some who participated in the two-year struggle for a medical education bill, may have been purposely exacerbated by those who wanted no bill at all. The issue seems one on which reasonable men might disagree: the prestigious schools wanted the basis of federal aid to be financial need; the have-less schools would get less aid if greater emphasis were not placed on incentive money for increased enrollments. But if such disagreement might be the natural result of differing needs and perspectives, all parties to the original formula knew how carefully the plan had been worked out, how delicate the coalition was. Thus, the "conspiratorial theory" goes, the problem with the Russell-Kerr amendment was that some favoring it didn't want federal aid in the first place; that controversy was consciously attached to the bill by a simple amendment which, on the surface, smacked only of the natural desire of some of the people's representatives to get more for their particular constituents.

The particular controversy over sustenance or expansion caused the medical schools' support to crumble. But whatever the medical deans did at that juncture may have been irrelevant. For Taft had changed his mind on the bill itself. He gave the Senate

> a general statement as to why I am opposed to this bill.
>
> Although I joined in the introduction of the bill, it seems to me that the conditions have entirely changed since the bill was drawn three years ago . . . the bill would add approximately $50,000,000 or $60,000,000 to the budget of the Government for the next 5 years.
>
> So far as I am concerned, I believe we have reached a point in the mobilization program where we cannot afford to undertake any new program unless emergency character can be shown beyond any question of doubt.
>
> . . . Every domestic expenditure is claimed to be for an emergency program. I do not see that it is . . . The only emergency I see is that more doctors are needed for the armed services. Any persons who start their education now will not be doctors for 6 years, so for the immediate emergency program this bill could be of no avail.
>
> . . . There is a provision for scholarships for doctors,

nurses and dentists. There is not the slightest emergency requirement for scholarships for doctors. There are more applications for entrance to medical schools than the schools can handle . . . There is no need for a scholarship program for dentists at the present time . . .

So far as the construction is concerned, I cannot see any more emergency in that regard than in the case of any other construction . . .

Therefore, I do not feel that there is anything in this bill which justifies the contention that it provides for an emergency which is related to the immediate building up of our mobilization strength against Russia.

. . . If we obligate ourselves to spend the money called for by this bill, the result will simply be to increase what we have to borrow from the American people and, therefore, to cause the inflation which will be brought about by such a procedure . . .

So it seems to me that we should strike out all of the bill except the part creating a committee to study the entire problem of medical education. Unless that is done, I shall oppose the bill and shall vote against it.[38]

Angered and feeling betrayed, Senator Pastore moved to recommit the bill to the Labor and Public Welfare Committee and the motion carried. The AMA's victory was won. Said Pastore:

Here I am. I was entrusted by the unanimous expression of the Committee with the management of the bill on the floor of the Senate, yet at the last moment, I find myself abandoned by those who participated in the hearings, and by those who had to do with the drafting of the bill . . . So my motive and reason for moving to recommit the bill was to send it back for further instructions to the same men who gave it to me to manage.[39]

Whether a more seasoned floor manager would have made the same move is a fair question. Republican Senator Edward Thye of Minnesota, who stood by the original bill, expressed surprise at the recommital motion.[40] Senator Taft gave his interpretation of Senator Pastore's move: "It was that he did not believe he had the votes, when the amendment was defeated, because he had offered it in order to get the votes of some of the southern Senators." [41]

Senator Willis Smith of North Carolina revealed, perhaps inadvertently, another factor in the bill's defeat:

> I was in favor of the bill, with one or two exceptions. One of the exceptions was that I did not want any bureaucrat in Washington to get control of the medical profession or of the medical schools . . .
>
> When I first read the bill, it did not concern me too much on that point, until I read the paragraph at the top of page 41, in large print. However, in small print, we find the following in the committee report: "Section 338 specifically prohibits Federal interference with or control over the curriculum or administration of any school or the admission of applicants thereto, except . . . in the few instances in which the bill carries specific requirements on this score." . . . Certainly we do not want the Federal Government to control who shall attend these schools.[42]

The alarming provision, to Senator Smith and other southern Senators, would have prevented scholarships from being denied on the basis of race, creed, or color and prevented admissions policies excluding out-of-state residents. William G. Reidy, long-time aid of Senator Murray and a key staff man on the bill, says that rumors of the bill's requiring the admission of northern Negroes to southern medical schools circulated in the Senate on the last day of the debate, and probably contributed to its defeat.[43]

Senator Homer Capehart (R., Ind.) unkindly suggested that "it looks like to me as though the able Senator from Rhode Island got caught in his own trap . . . He made a motion to recommit and it carried. He has all sorts of alibis . . . I appreciate the fact that he is new in the Senate and possibly did not realize what he was doing." [44] But Senator Hubert Humphrey said: "It is perfectly obvious that we did not have the votes to pass this measure, and it is for that reason that its recommital was recommended." [45]

The clearest reason for the bill's defeat was the AMA. It had helped defeat in the 1950 elections the principal proponent of the measure on the House side, Congressman Biemiller, and it saw itself as potential king-maker in the presidential elections of 1952. Later, it claimed to have been solely responsible for General Eisenhower's election—a claim the then President did not take kindly to despite presidential-AMA agreements on several items. But the Association would really have preferred Senator Taft to be President. And Senator Taft was very anxious to have the AMA's backing.

Senator Kerr needled Taft about his presidential ambitions in mock acceptance of Taft's stated reasons for changing his position on the bill: "Mr. President, I am sure that my friend the Senator from Ohio will be in the Senate for a number of years, and I am sure that he is not interested in any other campaign for a number of years, and therefore I am sure that what would cause the Senator from Ohio to arrive at that conclusion is a general philosophy on his part rather than a consideration of any approaching election." [46]

The nearest thing to an endorsement of Taft that the AMA could offer took place two months after the Senator had delivered the death blow to the medical education bill. Taft was one of two "most able and highly respected representatives of this country's major political parties" invited to address, before live television cameras, "a great, non-partisan forum" produced by the AMA in conjunction with the annual meeting of the

House of Delegates.[47] The representative of the Democratic Party was Senator Harry Byrd—who specified to the audience of 6,800 people, lest it not be understood: "I am a Jeffersonian Democrat of the old school . . . I am an anti-socialist Democrat, which means, in plain language, I am *not* a Truman Democrat."

Dr. John W. Cline, president of the AMA, who presided over the nonpartisan gathering, told the crowd that the two addresses they were to hear were a "highly significant preview of the major issues in The Great Debate of 1952." There was no covering up the fact that the audience would hear no real debate, and Dr. Cline did not try. "Each of our guests is completely free to say what he thinks on both domestic and international issues, but, knowing the character of these men, I am confident each of them will make his views clear on what we consider to be the key issue in America today—freedom versus socialism."

Elaborately praising Senator Taft in introducing him, Dr. Cline reminded the assembly that "his father was the 27th President of the United States," and he continued: "there are many who feel the son may follow in his father's footsteps. "

Taft, and of course Byrd, attacked socialism, which Taft defined as "the growing power of government in the affairs of all of you individuals, and its increased activity in many fields where it has never heretofore been involved." He praised the AMA for "taking the lead in opposing this trend," which, he said, "cannot be stopped, unless you are willing to elect both a President and a Congress who believe that the maintenance of liberty is the first and most essential consideration for progress."

The predictable speeches of that evening, December 15, 1951, were more than just a preview of "The Great Debate of 1952." They signaled past victories and continuing power, and foretold another decade of inaction on measures which many thought the nation needed, but which the American Medical Association vehemently opposed.

There was only one conceivable advantage for those concerned about advancing the cause of health. From a position of skeptical if largely unstated neutrality about the federal sponsorship of medical research—a position beginning with the incidental expression of concern in 1937 that establishment of the National Cancer Institute might trigger other like programs —the American Medical Association moved to an explicit, if cautious statement approving the principle involved. The Association itself was to remain outside the great national medical research enterprise, a fact not without irony; but one of the messages received during the battle of 1951 was that the AMA would at least not oppose the Congress if it moved to open up new fronts in the war it still wanted to wage, through research, against dread disease.

V   Emerging Congressional Leadership

The elements affecting the rise of the National Institutes of Health as the center of a new medical research empire between the war's end and the beginning of the Eisenhower Administration are so many and so diverse that it is hard even now to reconstruct them into a coherent whole. But that the strong foundation for such an empire was in place by January 1953 is clear: in seven years the NIH budget climbed from $7-plus million (in fiscal year 1947, the first full year of peace) to $70 million in the first year of Dwight D. Eisenhower's presidency.[1]

Looking at the phenomenon from this distance of time, it appears largely a matter of NIH filling a vacuum, or several vacuums. The American people were believed to be concerned about health as a national issue; but President Truman's plan to upgrade the nation's health and guarantee the availability of proper medical care to all citizens became so controversial that the only channels remaining open for federal health initiatives were those of facilities construction and research. Government leaders and statesmen of the science world wanted to build a system of support and coordination, by government, of science and research, including medical research; but failure to reach a consensus on central principles for five years led important public and private figures, some of their appetites whetted by popular interest as well as by personal and political needs, to embrace the National Institutes of Health as the main vehicle for government involvement in medical research. Thus was limited experience chosen over total freshness.

If in large measure NIH-national medical research growth resulted from the aggregate condition that scientific talent, political interest, popular concern, hence federal dollars had no place else to go, there are other factors that should not be forgotten. One is that in the first years of great expansion, one political party controlled the executive branch and the other the legislative.

Congress and the executive branch often seem to work at cross purposes regardless of party control. Students of the American party system may attribute such inevitable tensions to the existence of congressional and presidential branches of both the Democratic and Republican parties, each with its own needs, purposes, and plans. Still, no one doubts that a president's chances of seeing his policy prerogatives and program proposals, and his budget, remain intact are considerably greater when his party controls Congress; and that those chances are lessened when it does not.

Republican capture of the Eightieth Congress in the elections of 1946 signaled, in a dramatic way, the end of the bipartisan wartime coalition on a great range of issues. It gave warning that partisanship was once again fair play. The parties renewed the ancient battle, challenging each other over issues old and new and vying mightily over new program initiatives. In the case of medical research policy and the building of NIH, what later came to be advertised and accepted as a nonpartisan or bipartisan cause had some of its origins in precisely that partisan situation.

The House of Representatives

The National Institutes of Health began asking for more money after waking up to the realization that Congress was in a generous mood and looking for good new bets. Spurred on by the reassurances of friends and the fear of potential rivals, NIH got approval to ask Congress for $23 million in 1947 for fiscal year 1948; it received from Congress $26.5 million, over three times as much as the year before when the Democrats were in control, and over $3 million more than the President had requested. Congress so acted because the Republican chairmen of the appropriations subcommittees overseeing the NIH budget,

Congressman Frank Keefe of Wisconsin and Senator Edward Thye of Minnesota, argued that the national interest required it.

The precedent was cast in terms of a different struggle—the executive versus the legislative, rather than the Republicans versus the Democrats—but the partisan element was there. It was a precedent that was followed in most years to come, even when both Congress and the executive were controlled by the Democrats; and it was followed with a vengeance in that period in the fifties when the 1948 situation was reversed and a Republican president had to cope with a Democratic Congress.

There are other indications that party affiliation has, over the years, influenced decisions on medical research spending levels if not on policy generally.[2] Despite these occasional evidences of partisanship, and even evidence that sometimes the grand strategy over control of the medical research enterprise has been grounded in party loyalties, always on the surface and often in truth the cause of medical research has been nonpartisan.

In any case, Frank Keefe's goals were not essentially partisan even if his 1947 tactics were. One of his goals was much less grand than that of trying to seize policy initiative from the executive branch: he simply wanted to retain supervisory direction over medical research within the subcommittee he chaired. Hence he could play, and did, a liberal role if the challenge to his position as "health research leader" came from the outside in the form of a restrictive executive budget; or he could, in the traditional fashion of earlier congressional friends of the Public Health Service, play a more conservative role if special promoters inside Congress or the committee tried to foist new activities on those directly in charge.

Members of Congress whom the Public Health Service-National Institutes of Health considered friends in the prewar days were those who mainly staved off proposed "radical departures"—usually involving new health goals, enlarged budgets, expanded activities—by would-be friends who, for PHS tastes, were much too zealous. Thus Senator Ransdell was called upon by PHS officials to check the cancer plan of Senator Neely in the twenties; Senator Bone was encouraged to propose a more moderate, less threatening (to bureaucratic control) plan for cancer research than Congressman Maverick had in mind in the thirties. With an indomitable Matt Neely back in Congress in the forties, Frank Keefe was one of those counted upon to help keep things in the road—the middle of the road.

> Representative Keefe: The question arises in my mind as to whether or not we should allow an emotional appeal to overemphasize, perhaps, the realities at issue in this matter. I am wondering whether or not the mere appropriation of money and an enlargement of the program in some way, by giving it sudden impetus or push with a large shot of money is, in effect, going to produce the research that all of us hope will provide a cure for cancer . . . After all is said and done, there must be some reasonable limitation on the number of research people you can find . . . There is a limitation, is there not?
>
> Dr. Dyer: Certainly there is a limitation. The limitation comes about probably more from the somewhat limited number of trained personnel and men who can be attracted to the field. Men who have originality of ideas in addition to training.[3]

Keefe was already in a position of unparalleled influence over medical research, stemming from institutional authority: in 1944 the Public Health Service had become that rare agency authorized on a continuing basis to spend funds for certain purposes, in this case research, with no fixed ceiling.[4] Congress still has to decide annually how much money it can, and wants to, make available for the coming year, but the burden of securing annual authorizations as well as annual appropriations was thus removed. Formal, official policy was, in short, to "conquer cancer and other dread diseases"; implementation of that policy —itself a part of policy—would, on the legislative side of government, be left up to the House and Senate Appropriations Committees.

Congressional decisions on which most government activities are begun or continued occur in what is usually a painfully slow, 18-step process. Decisions are made or reviewed by two sub-committees, two full committees, two houses of Congress, a conference committee which must reconcile any differences in the actions of the two houses, and finally, in the first phase, two further deliberations by the House and the Senate on the decision of the conference committee. And that's only the authorization process. A similar mazurka follows to produce the actual dollars. No wonder informal practices have been developed to smooth the procedure; one of them is simply that the parent committee usually defers to the subcommittee's decisions on program content, scale, or proposed appropriation.

Still, to reduce that process by half is a singularly happy blessing for the agency in question. To eliminate the annual authorization process is also a blessing to the appropriation subcommittee chairman, if only because he does not have to wait until the legislative committee acts first, as it must according to the usual protocol. And if the subcommittee appropriation chairman has ideas of his own about the way in which, or the level at which, programs ought to be operated, such an arrangement gives him a near-exclusive franchise on the activity.

Whatever Frank Keefe's tactical motives might have been during his chairmanship of the Labor-Federal Security Subcommittee, his commitment to medical research was genuine. It probably did not hurt that Mary Lasker, also a native of Wisconsin, encouraged him and that Mr. Lasker had important business interests in the state; and Keefe certainly did not think he was engaged in an unpopular cause. He told his new friend Florence Mahoney that he had only one speech on the campaign trail, and that it was on health and what the federal government must do to advance it. That speech got him elected to five consecutive terms in Congress.

Keefe's daughter complained that he talked about health and medical research even at dinner.[5] And he got annoyed if other members of his committee did not evidence the interest he thought medical research deserved. When a member of the opposite party sat reading the newspaper one day during testimony on the NIH budget, Keefe banged his gavel: "Mr. Fogarty," he said, "this is important business we're considering here; you ought to pay attention and maybe you'll learn something." [6]

Democratic Congressman John Fogarty of Harmony, Rhode Island, had paid closer attention when the Labor Department's budget was being considered. That was what he was interested in, being a product and representative of the labor movement. He gave no sign, however, of being a "budget-raiser" even for the Labor Department. If he had, he probably would never have been assigned to that subcommittee.

Among the "norms," the unwritten rules that govern the House Appropriations Committee's approach to the public purse, is that which is supposed to preclude big spenders from committee membership.[7] Traditionally, the House Appropriations Committee considers its proper function that of cutting budgets submitted by the executive branch. Under the chairmanship of Clarence Cannon of Missouri, who ruled the Committee for decades, that norm seemed elevated to the level of a biblical commandment.

As a corollary to the rule, chairman Cannon, his colleagues report, would seldom assign a committee member to any subcommittee reviewing appropriations in which the member manifested any special interest. But as in the case of presidents and their Supreme Court appointees, committee chairmen can never be certain of the future performance of their subcommittee designees.

Fogarty became chairman of the Labor-Federal Security Agency appropriations subcommittee in January 1949, as a result of Harry Truman's having run successfully for re-election not just against Governor Dewey but, as well, against the "Republican, do-nothing 80th Congress." If Fogarty's several years' service on the subcommittee had primed him for the job it was not apparent as he presided over his first budgetary hearings in that same month. He was not always present for the hearings, occasionally leaving the second-ranking Democrat on the Committee, Representative E. H. Hedrick, M.D., from West Virginia, in charge.[8] Whoever officially presided over the hearings, Mr. Keefe of Wisconsin dominated them. Fogarty did not mind; he was in fact still learning from Keefe, more avidly than ever now that he was chairman. On more than one occasion Fogarty told the House that "there is not a Member of the House who knows more about the public health program of this country than does the gentleman from Wisconsin." [9]

Master lessons from Keefe to which Fogarty paid particular attention included procedural ones: first, Congress and its committees have a right to know what budgets professional agency heads think are necessary; second and similarly, Congress must not allow the Bureau of the Budget to deflect the impact of congressional initiatives of policy goals by reducing budgets unnecessarily; and third, subcommittee chairmen must have the backing of the ranking members of the opposite party, and preferably have unanimous committee reports if they are to do anything other than automatically reduce budget estimates submitted to their subcommittees. Implicit in all of this was the rule that health programs, and especially medical research and disease control programs, were never to be presented as partisan matters (even if committee members tended to divide along party lines as regards spending levels). The Budget Bureau was attacked not because it spoke for a Democratic administration against plans of a Republican congressman, but simply because it spoke for *the* administration against *a* congressional policy scheme. Fogarty observed how Keefe got away with increasing some budgets by reducing others. And he soon learned, from another source, that the committee chairmanship could bring campaign funds.

Keefe was shocked to learn in January 1949 that the Mental Health Division of the Public Health Service had been denied funds for construction of a facility on the NIH "campus" in Bethesda which Congress the previous year—when he chaired the subcommittee—had provided money for because such a facility was considered central to any effort to reduce mental illness. Chairman Fogarty too was surprised, saying: "As I remember the hearings of this committee over the last two years they placed a lot of emphasis on this construction."

Keefe's recollection was more precise: "I think it may be said that that was the very considered action of the subcommittee and of Congress itself . . . I thought Congress spoke in no uncertain terms as to what they wanted to see done. I am rather shocked at this time to see what I consider to be the ultimate guts of this program desecrated in this way by this august body we call the Bureau of the Budget." [10]

As to the second lesson, Keefe asked the associate director of NIH, Dr. Norman Topping, to tell the committee "how much you submitted to the Federal Security Agency, as one of its constituent agencies, as an estimate to carry out the full needs of NIH in 1950." [11]

Dr. Topping quoted the figures which NIH, with FSA approval, had asked for from the Budget Bureau. But that was not what Keefe wanted. He had, he said, figures suggesting that NIH could effectively spend about $30 million in fiscal 1950; what, then, would be the result of the agency's receiving only what it was now formally requesting?

> I know full well that you gentlemen are here to justify, pursuant to rules of procedure in appearing before congressional committees, the budget estimates submitted by the Bureau of the Budget. I believe the Committee and the Congress have an interest in knowing and understanding what the men who are charged with the responsibility of carrying out this service think and what their attitude is

as to what effect this budget allowance of $11.8 million is going to have out there at Bethesda.

Topping replied that it would certainly not allow the pace of in-house research to continue on schedule. What else, Keefe wanted to know? Topping thought of research grants and fellowships that would be discussed later. Keefe said, "Why not discuss it right now? That is what I am asking you. I am opening the door wide open to you without reservation and would expect you to give us the full and complete story."

Chairman Fogarty, catching on, then asked: "For the sake of the record, Doctor, will you follow these various programs and tell us in each case how much you asked the Bureau of the Budget for?" Later, he began to ask for "professional estimates": estimates made by each Institute Director and submitted to the "central office" at NIH.

That year the subcommittee reported to the House: "The committee made several reductions in budget items for the Public Health Service and at the same time has exceeded the estimates of four programs where the committee is convinced beyond a shadow of a doubt it is in the public interest to do so." [12]

Items increased over the budget estimates were: the National Cancer Institute, up $4 million; National Heart Institute, up $3.2 million; mental health division, up $2 million.

Senator Dennis Chavez of New Mexico, Fogarty's counterpart in the Senate, also recognized the popularity of medical research. Indeed he not only recognized it, he dramatized it, arranging for testimony by a variety of impressive figures, including some of Mrs. Albert Lasker's friends, on the need to expand our national medical research effort. Those who testified included James Adams, a reorganizer of the American Cancer Society with the Laskers and now chairman of the Society's executive committee; Dr. Paul Dudley White, the famous heart specialist; Dr. T. Duckett Jones, of equal renown; and others.

Senator Pepper asked to appear, to urge liberal appropriations for all health programs. In 1950 author John Gunther appeared before the Chavez committee to tell of his 17-year-old son's death from cancer. The Senate committee raised the appropriation for the Cancer Institute and for other institutes as well. Then the Senate itself, spurred by Senators Magnuson and Neely, raised the cancer budget still higher.[13] The total budget for the National Institutes of Health, as a result of renewed congressional interest and emerging congressional leadership, climbed to the record level of $50-plus million, almost twice what it had been the previous year. (The regular annual appropriation was $46.4 million; a supplemental appropriation raised the total to $52.1, according to the Office of Financial Management of NIH, or $51.5, according to figures compiled by Mary Lasker.)

1950 was a vortical year for medical research policy. Events of several years had led to the tentative, tacit acceptance of the National Institutes of Health as the major vehicle through which the federal government would seek to achieve policy goals. In 1950 that trend might conveniently have been turned around, because Congress and the executive branch seemed at long last to be reaching an understanding about the National Science Foundation. The new foundation might have been given jurisdiction over biomedical science and research; or, NIH might have been explicitly designated as the agency assigned the job of attacking disease, through research, on a wide front.

As usual, however, policy decisions were not so clearcut. The National Science Foundation, created by the law signed by President Truman in May 1950, contained a Division of Biological and Medical Sciences. Meanwhile, Congress in the same year passed the Omnibus Medical Research Act, which not only authorized establishment of the Institute of Neurological Diseases and Blindness and the Institute of Arthritis and Metabolic Diseases, but gave the Surgeon General authority to establish additional institutes, as he determined the need for them, to "conduct and support research and research training relating to other diseases and groups of diseases." [14]

In offering distinctions as between the goals of NSF's Medical Research Division and those of NIH, the director of the Science Foundation later said: "The National Institutes of Health stresses research aimed at the care and cure of diseases, including basic research related to its mission . . . The National Science Foundation, on the other hand, supports basic research in this area primarily for the purpose of advancing our knowledge and understanding of biological and medical fields." [15]

In short, the question of whether there should be a research foundation with a medical division or a separate medical research foundation—the question on which Dr. Bush and his designated study chairman disagreed, President Truman seemed ambivalent, and Mrs. Mahoney and Mrs. Lasker changed their minds depending on which option seemed at the time most promising—was settled (or allowed to settle) by doing both. Or, as Dr. Alan Waterman, then director of NSF, put it in 1960: "Actually, both recommendations have been met by subsequent events." [16]

NIH was not, then, to be the federal government's exclusive agent for medical research. The National Science Foundation was to have some role. Further, the Atomic Energy Commission was directed by Congress to look into the possibility of relating atomic research to cancer cure; $5 million was provided for the purpose in 1950.[17] And the Veterans Administration, which between the two world wars performed no research even in conjunction with its hospitals, had begun to enter the premises. The Defense Department, through its service medical branches, continued to probe for answers to medical problems, especially those relating to military situations.

Failure to make exclusive policy choices does not necessarily mean absence of policy. Retaining multiple options may be a conscious decision. Even if not fully coordinated, decisions may aggregate in such a way as to constitute policy, especially if those decisions do not, as they are executed, actually (though they may theoretically) conflict.

National medical research policy, as it gradually evolved in the postwar years, included the following elements accepted by the executive, Congress, the bureaucracy, and specialized interest groups: the federal government would support both basic and targeted research; it would support both through the National Institutes of Health, though the main concern there should be the conquest of specific diseases; it would also support targeted research through agencies having missions inviting special attention to particular problems; and it would provide for the support of basic, nontargeted biological and biomedical research through the National Science Foundation.

The logic of the arrangement no doubt seems clearer in retrospect than it did at the time, if indeed the arrangement itself seemed clear at the time. There were, of course, defenses to be offered of the essential overlapping of the purposes of the National Science Foundation and the National Institutes of Health. A popular one was: "With more than one source of funds available from the Federal Government scientists enjoy the broader base of support that is consistent with American tradition." [18] What was also consistent with American tradition was that the provision of a broad base of support from several sources was not a decision purposefully arrived at, but simply a phenomenon that occurred in the absence of a specific resolution of the issue.

Regardless of not being given exclusive designation as the government's prime mover on the medical research front, NIH had maneuvered itself—and been maneuvered—into just such a position. Using the authority given him (at his request) in the same year that the Science Foundation was established, Surgeon General Leonard Scheele created two new institutes, bringing the total number of institutes (and disease fields covered) to eight. NIH was given more than $50 million that year (fiscal 1951). It was going to attack arthritis, blindness and other diseases it thought important. It had not only saved itself from effective competition, but it had seized the policy initiative from the Congress. Or so it thought.

For its part, Congress was delighted with the new aggressive attitude of the agency. It was glad to go along with top officials who seemed to want to move out and do things. But Congress had no intention of now taking a back seat. It had brought the National Institutes of Health to the fore, had decided to make its heaviest commitment to medical research through the Institutes, and it wanted cancer conquered and other dread diseases eradicated.

The future looked good for medical research, and particularly for NIH, when the decade of the 1950's began; but the halcyon days did not immediately arrive. Once more, war interrupted.

From 1939 to 1969 appropriations for the National Institutes of Health climbed with some regularity. Although the Congress occasionally reduced particular NIH appropriations figures from those proposed, the only actual retrogression in the sequence of annual budget increases occurred in war years: in 1941 (FY42) and 1951 (FY52) the budget was reduced, and in 1967 (FY1968) it increased only marginally.

There is no surprise in the fact that heavy increases in national military and defense budgets are likely to produce simultaneous reductions in a whole range of domestic budgets. Lyndon Johnson tried mightily to destroy that seemingly inevitable rule in the mid-sixties but with scant success. Yet war can serve as a good excuse for not doing what one probably wouldn't do anyway. Senator Robert Taft used the Korean War and its impact on the budget as an excuse for changing his position favoring federal aid to medical schools; the real reason would seem to be that the American Medical Association changed its position and persuaded Taft to alter his.

In any event, the fiscal and political climates were not right for increasing medical research appropriations in 1951 and 1952, even though the new chairman of the House Appropriations Subcommittee did his best, spurred on by the ranking subcommittee member, Frank Keefe. Both thought the budget estimates presented by the agency were retrogressive, but other members of the subcommittee considered them more than adequate. For once, the usually all-powerful combination of committee chairman and ranking opposite party member could not get the rest of their colleagues to agree with them. And whenever there is such a split in appropriations committees, regardless of what the issue is, there is only a fair chance that the chairman will be upheld when the issue comes before the whole House. It is for this reason that the "norm of subcommittee unity," elaborated on by Richard Fenno as a cohesive force in congressional appropriations committees, actually works. It is for this reason that unanimous, bipartisan reports are the goal of every appropriations subcommittee chairman, and it is why the chairmen are often willing to compromise their own positions in order to attain the goal.[19]

Keefe's Republican colleague on the subcommittee, Everett P. Scrivener, had been uncomfortable when the ranking member had castigated the Budget Bureau during the fiscal 1951 hearings. He thought the Bureau did good work, he said. And he was unsure whether adding dollars to the NIH budget would really hasten results.

> As much as we are sold on research, there is still a limit on what we can do. These programs keep climbing, and it is easy to see why the budget keeps going up and up . . . We seem to be running into a never ending series of increased requests. If this were the only program the Government were carrying on it would be simple, but before every Appropriation Subcommittee sitting today that same thing is taking place. Everyone wants more for their particular agency.[20]

Congressman Christopher Columbus McGrath (D., N.Y.) agreed.[21] Apparently Fogarty and Keefe couldn't bring the two around. The result was that Keefe decided to carry amendments to the floor to increase medical research appropriations. Though Fogarty supported him, dozens of his colleagues praised him for his leadership in health and research, and he pulled all dramatic stops, climaxing his plea with the revelation that he did not intend to seek re-election to the Eighty-second Congress, Keefe—and NIH—lost.[22] The triple handicap—violating the appropriations committee norm of upping rather than cutting budgets, having to appeal to the House over objections of a majority of his committee colleagues, and attempting all of this in time of war and the accompanying "tighten the domestic belt" theme—proved insurmountable.

It was 1952 before the medical research budget started moving upward again. The upturn in that year was spurred by Senator Chavez, although Congressman Fogarty was able to get the House to approve a budget figure for NIH closer to the Senate's proposed appropriation than what it had adopted originally. Fogarty's success in this respect was significant for the future, for it spotlighted an important juncture in the sequential pattern that produced consistent congressional increases in medical research budgets for years to come.

That the Senate is lightly referred to as the "upper body," because it is prone to increase appropriations figures over those approved by the more conservative House, doesn't make House members feel any better about the frequency with which their serious work is ignored by their Senate colleagues. Hence it is not an automatic proposition that the House will accept an appropriations conference report containing amounts much higher than those it had accepted originally. It demands, in short, a selling job. Fogarty's salesmanship was impressive and became more so as time went on. His abilities grew with experience, and that is a good thing, for some of his colleagues became increasingly suspicious that he didn't argue hard enough in representing the House position in the conference committee; that he expected the other side to win the checker game, and that he didn't mind.

On his part, despite the fact that those who were unsure of the propriety or the advantage of increasing medical research budgets did seize upon the Korean War to slow that trend, Fogarty's selling ability was aided by his conviction that medical research was a popular as well as a viable endeavor, hence one that, politically, was difficult to oppose.

In 1953 he had a perfect chance to test that thesis. He had had to give up his chairmanship when President Eisenhower's coattails brought a majority of Republicans into Congress. The Republican House majority was small, however: 221 Republicans to 213 Democrats and one independent. Calculating the factors of that small majority, the inexperience of the new chairman (Fred Busbey of Illinois), and the "tradition" of bipartisan support based on wide public appeal, ranking subcommittee member John Fogarty moved on the floor that the House increase the Administration's proposed budget for the National Institutes of Health, despite the committee's formal acceptance of the figures in that budget.

Obviously the challenge was as much or more to Chairman Busbey as it was to President Eisenhower, but Fogarty was gentle with the Gentleman from Illinois. "Mr. Chairman," he said, addressing the presiding officer of the Committee of the Whole House, "I think we have a pretty good bill this year, though I think there are some places where we [on the Appropriations Committee] have cut too much." [23] Or not added enough, he might have said. His colleague, Antonio Manuel Fernandez of New Mexico, the only other Democrat on the subcommittee, supported him: "I think we have come here with a fair bill, and if we can make it a little more adequate tomorrow [when we take up amendments] we will still be happier. I want to associate myself with the views of my good friend from Rhode Island in respect to the various increases [he has suggested]." [24]

Chairman Busbey had also pondered some of the factors Fogarty had, and before the Fogarty amendments increasing budgets for various medical research activities could be voted on, Busbey accepted them, insuring their automatic adoption by the House.[25] Thus was an additional $5 million given to NIH by the House.

With similar party numbers prevailing in the Senate (49 Republicans and 47 Democrats) and with a generally sympathetic subcommittee chairman, Edward Thye, the Senate friends of medical research added over $10 million more to the House figure.[26] The amount the conference committee had agreed to was close to the amount voted by the Senate—$71 million, $10 million more than Fogarty had gotten the House to agree to in the first round—and now Fogarty got the House to accept that figure. His thesis had proved correct, and he reinforced it with similar results in 1954. Now began in earnest the congressional effort to take charge of the medical research enterprise and make it its own, an effort made somewhat easier when the Democrats regained control of Congress in the elections that fall.

One of the central planks in John Fogarty's re-election platform was that of improving the nation's health through medical research.

The Senate

In a decision he later said he regretted[27] Senator Chavez, a Democrat, decided not to reassume chairmanship of the subcommittee handling health appropriations when the Democrats organized the Eighty-fourth Congress (1955–56). Instead he chose the chairmanship of the Defense Appropriations Subcommittee.

That Senator Lister Hill would succeed to the chairmanship Chavez left seems only natural now, but at the time it was not automatic. For one thing, the same subcommittee controlled education budgets. And federal aid to education had, with Supreme Court's school desegregation decision of 1954,[28] become an issue that Hill, with his Alabama constituency seething resentment against "Washington," would have much preferred to stay away from. Personally, he was strongly in favor of federal expenditures for education, just as he had always been for federal aid in building hospitals and rural electrification systems and dams. Subsequently, he devised a strategy to insure safe passage through his Committee on Labor and Public Welfare, between 1955 and 1969, of more federal education aid provisions than anyone had thought possible; and this during a period when other southern Democrats were using all the traditional power their committee chairmanships provided to block federal aid on a number of fronts, especially those where federal involvement might mean federal pressure to eliminate segregation.

Hill's interest in health and medicine was a factor drawing him to the newly available chairmanship. The son of a physician who had pioneered in heart surgery (and named after his father's mentor, Lord Joseph Lister), with a number of close male relatives who were physicians, Lister Hill might also have become a doctor except for a critical barrier encountered at an early age: he became ill at the sight of open wounds.[29] He had already made a name for himself in the Senate in the health field by sponsoring that legislation in 1946 which marked the entry of the federal government into an important new area relating to the people's health: the Hill-Burton Hospital Construction Act.

Still, all these connections—later recited in one breath as if to suggest the inevitability of his emergent leadership in health—were not, at the time the key decision had to be made, overpowering. He had other interests after all (agriculture and military affairs, to name two), which, developed into an area of special expertise and influence, would have pleased the voters back home.

Florence Mahoney was afraid Hill might choose another role, might leave the health-education appropriations chairmanship to one of his colleagues. She used all her persuasive powers, now well developed after a decade in the legislative health arena, to convince him what the right decision was. He could, she told the Senator, become America's most prominent health states-man. It was clear the Eisenhower Administration was not pre-pared to do anything for the nation's health. And the principal issue needing attention, medical research, was noncontroversial. Indeed, Hill could become a national figure with national pres-tige.

Hill had given up on that possibility after 1948, when most of his fellow delegates from Alabama had walked out of the Dem-ocratic National Convention and his State had subsequently voted for Governor J. Strom Thurmond of South Carolina, can-didate of the States Rights Democratic (Dixiecrat) party, for president. Hill voluntarily resigned his position as Senate Dem-ocratic Whip and enhanced his efforts to shed the image, in Alabama, of the "New-Deal-Fair-Deal Democrat" that had been attached to him with some reason. In 1940 it had been Hill who nominated Franklin D. Roosevelt for a third term as president; in 1948 Hill mounted the rostrum at the Philadelphia convention to propose for president his colleague from Georgia, Senator Richard Brevard Russell. Hill's filibusters against every piece of civil rights legislation introduced in Congress in the post-Brown era were as long as any others'. But if he was a true believer in the States Rights Movement of the time, it was, to him, a limit-ing if not a lost cause.

In the final analysis, it was health that seemed right for Hill. He assumed chairmanship of the Subcommittee on Labor-Health, Education and Welfare Appropriations in January 1955. It was a date of extraordinary significance for medical research in the United States—and for Lister Hill. When he retired from the Senate 14 years later Hill was justly hailed as "Mr. Health." Some 60 health measures had become law under his sponsorship. His praises were elaborately sung by colleagues liberal and conservative upon his retirement, a fine tribute but a customary tradition; what was somewhat unusual, and not often occasioned by a congressional retirement, were the editorial praises of newspapers across the country including the *New York Times*.[30] Dennis Chavez might have been merely paying Hill a compliment when he said, in 1960, that he was sorry he had given up that chairmanship to Lister Hill. But on the other hand he might have been serious, for with it he gave up the chance to become one of the more celebrated men in public office in the United States.

As he took charge of the Senate effort to shape national medical research policy and build the size of the research effort, Senator Hill enjoyed greater advantages, politically and institutionally, than did Congressman Fogarty. Like Fogarty, Hill's immediate predecessor was a Republican who favored the medical research enterprise. Ed Thye of Minnesota had been considered a friend of the cause during his two years as chairman in the Eighty-third Congress (when he had succeeded Chavez), and he continued to be helpful as Hill's ranking opposite.

Thye's was a somewhat less zealous approach. This was partially because he was a Republican, in the judgment of Senator Hill and of Thye's Republican colleague Roman Hruska of Nebraska. Hruska acknowledges that both Republicans and Democrats who, like him and Thye, have served on the appropriations subcommittee have contributed to the rapid growth of the medical research enterprise; that both have contributed to its becoming known as a "congressional program." But, he suggests, while he and most of his Republican colleagues generally "went along" with certain increases in annual proposed budgets of NIH, they had been more discriminating while remaining progressive. Hill and the Democrats, in Hruska's view, were just plain extravagant.[31]

Hill's explanation of the situation is compatible with the main point, though it places the emphasis elsewhere. Thye was sympathetic, says Hill, but "afraid to go after big money." Senator Margaret Chase Smith, an early and consistent supporter of medical research, confirms the point.

In any case, despite differences in preferred amounts for increases in medical research appropriations, Thye's precedent as chairman and his continuing cooperation justified Hill's claim, like Fogarty's made religiously in introducing the annual appropriations measure to the parent house, that medical research was a bipartisan enterprise. Republicans and Democrats, liberals and conservatives on the committee all agreed, Hill reported with pious regularity to the Senate, that Congress must lead the nation forward, through research, into a Golden Age of Medicine. And that great national goal, toward which congressional policy was aimed, could only be attained by following the bipartisan plan of spending more now.

The advantage of bipartisanship, a strategic political advantage, was reinforced for Hill by Styles Bridges' senior position on the full Appropriations Committee. Bridges was influential with most Republicans and with all fiscal conservatives; and from the time Mrs. Lasker got him to sponsor the National Heart Act, in 1948, she remained influential with him.

As if the institutional advantage of NIH appropriations being made without renewed authorization were not enough, Hill's other advantages included his succeeding to chairmanship of the Committee on Labor and Public Welfare in the same year he chose the health appropriations subcommittee. In the House of Representatives, legislative committee chairmen, not infrequent enthusiasts for programs appertaining to their domains, frequently meet grief at the hands of their appropriations committee counterparts. By the same token, he whose role it is to control the proceeds of the public purse usually finds in the fervent legislative committee chairman-sponsors of given programs the bane of his purser's existence. In the Senate, where in contrast to the House membership on the Appropriations Committee does not preclude membership on other important committees, such likely conflicts between committees and committee chairmen are not built into the legislation-appropriation process. Still, rare is the opportunity for a single senator to be able to write legislation that launches programs and then to control the pace of their progress by insuring provision of the necessary funds. Such, beginning in 1955, was Hill's good fortune.

There was yet another boon that Hill capitalized on in positioning the medical research enterprise for its subsequent spectacular flight. The chairman of the Senate Appropriations Committee, Carl Hayden (D., Ariz.), was not only permissive but almost always supportive of his subcommittee chairmen.[32] Indeed, rarely has so much congressional power gone so unexploited as that which Hayden potentially held as chairman of the Senate Appropriations Committee. The beloved old man from Arizona was said to be so deferential to his subcommittee chairmen that he was reluctant to ask for the least favor. Naturally an effort was made to meet any of his needs or desires that might be divined by his juniors on the committee. But his benign rule of many years stands out in sharp contrast to the ways of other committee chairmen.

John Fogarty, meanwhile, having himself shown insufficient reverence for the norm of relentless budget-cutting, was hardly surprised—despite his occasional public expression of that reaction—that his full committee chairman, Clarence Cannon (D., Mo.), did not approve the Labor-HEW subcommittee's proposed appropriation levels for medical research. The total amounts for all agencies were usually below the budget estimates of the executive branch, but the proposed figure for NIH was almost always higher than the budget proposal. Cannon did not like exceptions to the rule, especially when the one in question seemed to be developing into a permanent exception. He not only took advantage of his ex officio position on all subcommittees and came to "markup sessions" of the subcommittee, but when final figures were decided upon he often brought his ranking opposite, the equally conservative John Taber of New

York, with him—an intimidating congressional combination if there ever was one. Except, it should be added, to John Fogarty.

Executive branch officials watched with incredulity, even dismay, as Congress began to take over the matter of fixing the medical research budget almost without regard to the Administration's budget estimates set by the Bureau of the Budget. From 1950 through 1953 (fiscal 1951–1954) the Budget Bureau annually proposed an increase of $1 million in the NIH budget, a regular incremental advance in the finest BOB tradition. The Congress in that period fluctuated in its reaction, affected by wars and political situations, sometimes cutting and sometimes adding but not proceeding on any fixed schedule such as the executive obviously preferred. Not that an extra million dollars a year didn't seem like plenty in the eyes of some House pursers. Representative Taber agreed with the budget-makers downtown: "It seems to me, Mr. Chairman, that when we give an increase of $1 million over last year's appropriation we are doing as much as we ought to do at this time. You cannot appropriate a lot of extra money to any one of these agencies and have them absorb it efficiently at any given time." [33]

There had been a time in the rather recent past when the NIH itself would have agreed. Now, however, it seemed to enjoy the attention given, and the dollars lavished, by its congressional sponsors.

For the first three years of the Eisenhower Administration, Congress regularly added anywhere from $8 to $15 million to the proposed NIH budget; and the first two of those years, the President's own party held a majority in (if they did not in the strict sense "control") the Congress. The Administration response in the first two years was to suggest budgets in lesser amounts than the previous year's congressional appropriations. Somehow, the executive had not got the message of congressional desires and intentions.

The first Secretary of Health, Education and Welfare, Mrs. Oveta Culp Hobby, gave no indication of recognizing the implications this developing pattern held for executive management; but the Undersecretary of HEW, Nelson Rockefeller, did.[34] He was particularly annoyed at the technique chairman Fogarty used to make NIH officials reveal what they had asked for originally; and at the ease, it seemed to him, with which they backslid from defense of the Administration budget. On one occasion Rockefeller severely scolded an NIH official after a House subcommittee hearing. Word quickly got back to the chairman, who, in addition to publicly expressing his wrath about the Undersecretary's actions, which he equated with an attempt to prevent the Congress from getting the whole truth, suggested that he intended to cut the budget of the Secretary's Office.

Nor did it seem to help the Administration regain a semblance of control over the medical research budget to raise that particular controversy to a philosophical level. Rockefeller stated his position as follows:

> My philosophy is that everything possible should be done for the health of this Nation but that there is more than one group that is servicing the health of the Nation. It is not only the Federal Government. It is the Federal, State, and local governments, and these tremendous private organizations . . . throughout the country . . . We have got to gear in and mesh into the total picture and let the Federal Government play the part which it is right for it to play.

And Fogarty stated his: "I do not think we are going far enough. I think we should be doing more than we are doing . . . The Federal Government could do more than it is doing at the present time and accomplish results by spending money."[35]

There seemed to be no turning Fogarty and his zealous congressional colleagues around. It seemed to be that, as Fogarty's erstwhile colleague and onetime chairman, Fred Buseby, had put it: "you will support any program that increases appropriations." Fogarty admitted it: "As long as it helps to save lives I positively will, and I do not care how much it costs . . . If it is going to save lives or if it is going to help solve the health problems of this country, I am not going to quibble whether it is $25 million or $100 million." [36] With Fogarty's energetic help, the NIH budget came within calling distance of the $100 million the following year, 1956.

What was developing was, in the phrase of one who watched the process at close range, a baronial power league where treaties and contracts and grants were drawn up in utter disregard of the rules of the monarchy. Notwithstanding their traditional obligations, the fealty of NIH officials was to those most concerned with their interests. And those interests had become expansionist.

Dr. William Sebrell, who was director of NIH from 1950 to 1955, stated his attitude, including his acceptance of the dominant congressional role in the league, when he testified before the Fogarty committee in 1954: "I am not going to violate the wishes of Congress. If Congress says that they want the bulk of the money spent on cancer or neurology, or what have you, then that is where the money is going, insofar as I am concerned." [37]

Dr. Leonard Scheele may have been the last happy Surgeon General of the Public Health Service. He had been unafraid of the new medical research lobby, or that congressional friends of the medical research cause might "get out of control." Indeed, he thought a little boom period might be good for the enterprise, for he too had chafed under the rigidly conservative scientific approach of the microbiologists who, for most of its life, had set the pace of the National Institutes of Health and its predecessor organization. He not only verbally welcomed the support of an outside interest group; he helped elevate that group's importance and their influence by appointing them to policy advisory roles, in fact, by institutionalizing their role. He did not feel threatened by what others considered political intrusion into the scientific domain, or legislative trespassing onto executive turf; he seemed instead to favor it. What is perhaps more impressive and unusual, Dr. Scheele unabashedly encouraged the growth of one of the bureaus under his organizational jurisdiction despite increasing signs that it would soon dominate the entire agency and become so independent as to be uncontrollable by him who formally sat at the top of the organizational chart.

Medical research had not quite reached that status in the days that Dr. Scheele lavished public praise on the Congress for its prescient sponsorship of the effort. But it was clearly coming. The only thing needed, in Scheele's judgment, to insure that the enterprise grew soundly as it grew inevitably larger was a man of vision and strength, a scientist who was not just a manager but a planner. He selected as director of the National Institutes of Health Dr. James A. Shannon, a physician and physiologist whose research work in malaria during the war had earned him the Presidential Medal of Merit and who, before coming to the National Institutes of Health in 1952 (as associate director of the Heart Institute), had directed the Squibb Institute of Medical Research. Shannon became Director of NIH on August 1, 1955.

With the new NIH head a protégé, the medical research lobbyists his supporters, and John Fogarty a private heart patient, Scheele felt confident of his ability to move that medical research effort under his formal control toward the goals and at the pace he chose. But he was soon to depart the scene. His successors had increasingly less to say about what NIH did, and by 1968 the Surgeon General had been removed from the line of authority between NIH and the Secretary of Health, Education and Welfare.

Scheele had been appointed by President Truman to replace Dr. Parran mainly because Truman wanted to name "his own man"; he had been reappointed by President Eisenhower to the surprise of some, especially those unaware that he had worked for General Eisenhower in Europe. Scheele retired in the summer of 1956. From that point on, although the organizational chart remained the same, the director of NIH seemed to answer to nobody but Congress. Or as Dr. Shannon would prefer to put it, he *explained* matters to Congress.

Insuring the scientific integrity of the national medical research effort was one important matter. Insuring, if it were possible to do so, that the expenditure of federal funds did not totally escape executive jurisdiction was another. And if Secretary Hobby did not know how to cope with the problem, her successor thought he might.

On the same day that Shannon became the new NIH head, Marion B. Folsom became Secretary of Health, Education and Welfare. He came to the job immediately from the Treasury Department, where, since the start of the Eisenhower presidency, he had been Undersecretary to George Humphrey. It was not his service there so much as his earlier experience in helping set up the Social Security Administration that prompted the President to ask him to take the post; but his relationship with George Humphrey proved an enormous boon. Nor did it hurt that Folsom had, for a period during the war, headed up the staff of a committee of the House of Representatives on postwar planning and had made friends with the members of that committee, among them John Fogarty.[38]

On assuming his new post, Folsom found that the Department's budget for 1956 (fiscal 1957) had already been tentatively prepared. The President had been pleased with the small budget surplus of the previous year and wanted departmental budgets held at the same level for the coming year. It was assumed that anyone who had been a close associate of George Humphrey would be just the man to keep the budget down.

Two weeks after he had ensconced himself in his new office, Secretary Folsom had a telephone call from his old friend Anna Rosenberg, who wanted him to meet Mary Lasker. When they met, Folsom was impressed. He had rarely heard a woman argue a case so well. The case, of course, was for placing national medical research policy on a more important level of executive consideration than it had been; of viewing positively the possibilities that research held for improving the nation's health, rather than approaching the activity in the usual unimaginative, green-eye-shade manner. She reeled off statistics on mortality, illness, and debilitation, relating them to particular diseases; she described the state of the art in various research areas and specified particular research needs to meet certain timetables; she garnished this presentation of her knowledge of the state of biomedicine with figures on manpower and facilities. When she left, Folsom asked an assistant to check some of the figures Mrs. Lasker had proffered; when they were "verified" a few days later, he discovered that his staff member's source of verification was the Lasker group—apparently the only place where such data were compiled and correlated on a comprehensive scale.

Secretary Folsom shortly had another pair of visitors who were concerned about the medical research picture. Surgeon General Scheele and NIH Director Shannon came to protest the proposition of holding the medical research budget at the $100 million level for another year. To be so restricted, they said, would mean they would have to turn down grant applications from a number of excellent investigators whose proposed projects held real promise for medical advancement. In their judgment, to keep up a progressive pace the NIH budget should be increased by some $30 million.

Marion Folsom did not relish the idea that his first important move as Secretary of Health, Education and Welfare would be that of breaking the President's suggested budget ceiling. He did not, on the other hand, intend to approach his new job any more timidly than he had approached any other. He put together an ad hoc group of industrial researchers and laboratory directors, suggested by people he knew and trusted in the private research sector, and asked them to review NIH's projected needs and the quality of its work and operations. He was reassured on all counts.

Meanwhile, he determined that there were other serious

needs which the proposed budget of the Department could not accommodate, needs of a much greater scale than those of NIH. A congressional committee had recommended that, to rescue the medical schools from their perenially difficult financial plight, recently exacerbated by the Korean War, $50 million a year in matching grants for facilities construction ought to be committed for a five-year period. Folsom's private sources confirmed the need. And college classroom construction was lagging seriously; federal help was essential, according to those advising the Secretary. Folsom made a decision to secure approval of a budget figure that would accommodate all three budgetary additions.

In September 1955 President Eisenhower had a heart attack. From that point until his recovery, the Cabinet met frequently to discuss major issues. Presided over by Vice President Nixon, an appropriate Cabinet group was to reach consensus on important decisions, then transmit their recommendations to the President. Not all Cabinet members participated in the discussion of all issues, but George Humphrey had had an understanding with the President that he would be consulted on every matter that involved fiscal and monetary matters, in particular, government spending. Given that understanding and Humphrey's conservative approach and powerful personality, he was the fiscal terror of the administration.

One of Humphrey's keen interests in private life had been the Case University Medical School, in his home city of Cleveland; it was a source of pride to him that he had been elected to its board of trustees. Naturally it was not difficult to get Case to confirm the sad plight of medical schools generally, as well as its own situation. Further, Humphrey knew from experience that Marion Folsom was no easy man with a dollar. Yes, he would support the Secretary of Health, Education and Welfare in his proposal to the Cabinet that the HEW budget include at least an additional $80 million for medical school construction and medical research. With that blessing, the Cabinet approved.

Director of the Budget Percival Brundage, formerly a senior partner in the international accounting firm of Price, Waterhouse and Company, was considerably pained.

The President, whose condition was steadily improving, was meeting with his Cabinet officers one by one to review their programs and budgets for the coming year and other matters which they felt needed his attention. In November, Secretary Folsom's turn came to fly to Denver. He was delighted to find there Dr. Paul Dudley White, a strong champion of increased federal spending for medical research, attending the President. Whether Dr. White had been doing a little private presidential lobbying is not certain, but Folsom strongly suspects that he had; when Folsom told the President he wanted to increase the medical research budget by $30 million, Eisenhower's reaction was one of relief and immediate acceptance.

On the proposed new item for medical school construction—money which would go directly from the federal government to the qualified institution in need—the Secretary got an argument. The President wondered why such money could not be channeled through the States. Folsom replied that most medical schools were national in character, training young men and women who came from all over the country to be physicians, who would upon attaining their degrees practice medicine in various parts of the country, probably without regard to their geographical origins or where they had gone to medical school. There were a number of schools concentrated in certain states and regions, and other states had no medical schools. The national need could not be met by automatically channeling federal money through state mechanisms. Eisenhower accepted the argument.[39]

Jere Cooper of Tennessee, Democratic chairman of the House Ways and Means Committee, which didn't favor unrestricted spending for anything, thought President Eisenhower had made a splendid choice in selecting Marion Folsom for the HEW post. John Fogarty and Lister Hill, who favored liberal spending for medical research, thought so too. When Folsom appeared before their respective committees to present the fiscal 1957 budget, Hill and Fogarty acknowledged that he was the first Secretary who had demonstrated any understanding of medical research needs and possibilities, and of the relationship of the enterprise to the health and well-being of the country. For the first time, they said, the budget proposed by an Administration for NIH was in the ballpark of reality. They congratulated the Secretary on turning the trend around.

Secretary Folsom was pleased that they were pleased. "The House Committee on Appropriations," he reported to the Senate Committee, "in its introductory remarks in the report on the Appropriation bill was complimentary of the budget of the Department. It is gratifying to find that committee and the Department seeking basically the same objectives in carrying out the Federal role in areas of health, education and welfare. I believe there are fewer differences of view with respect to this budget than at any time in recent years." Senator Hill responded: "From the study I have given the budget, I think that is absolutely true; that the differences have been very much narrowed down from what they have been in past years, which is very pleasing, I might say." [40]

The Secretary soon discovered that turning around the executive budget approach as regards medical research needs was not the same thing as turning around the situation where the Congress led the way in suggesting program directions, or proposing modifications, or generally shaping policy, by deciding which research goals were most important to the country and at what speed they ought to be pursued.

Congressional interest in medical research, originally simple, even naive, inspired by dramatizations of mysteries of dread diseases and their imprint on friends, family, and colleagues, was becoming sophisticated and long-range. Congressional leadership—in the early days tentative, disjointed, and often highly personalized, assumed in the leadership vacuum left by the executive branch, sometimes spurred by partisan considerations and sometimes simply by the desire to build a personal record of compassionate public service—now had matured into a tradition which Congress was comfortable with and which it would not easily yield.

It was not that even key proponents of the Cause in Congress thought they knew enough to force medical research down fruitful paths which scientists were too dim to perceive. But they were less awestruck by medical doctors and biomedical scientists than in the early days. They had become convinced that the laboratory researcher's perspective was not the only view of what was scientifically important. They had discovered through experience that medical science, like other activities, was attracted to money, that the plentiful provision of dollars for specific research activities, new or old, would bring increased activity in those areas and, sometimes, productive results.

Just as Congress was less and less in awe of medical scientists and directors of biomedical research activities, it now ignored whatever proprieties may have obtained in given earlier periods regarding executive-legislative roles in setting specific policy directions and program goals. If there was an element of pride and rivalry in the congressional response to the Administration's medical research budget for 1957, still its main focus was on the medical research enterprise itself and what would bring it to the fullest and quickest success. And Congress might be forgiven, on the basis of its previous experience, if what the executive advanced as a progressive program did not meet congressional expectations on that score.

Senator Margaret Chase Smith, the Maine Republican who ordinarily supported her Republican President, simply thought it was about time the Administration stepped up the pace. "We haven't done too much in other years," she told the Secretary, "and except for the leadership of Senator Hill we wouldn't be doing what we are doing." [41] Senator Charles Potter (R., Mich.) agreed.[42] Senator Hill expressed surprise and simultaneous gratification; what he wondered was why the executive, after being so negative or at least so coy about what the Congress wanted to provide for medical research the previous year, had suddenly decided to put on a new face.

> Secretary Folsom came forth, very much certainly to my gratification, and I am sure to the gratification of other committee members and advised us that when he became Secretary last August he called in representatives of the NIH and other distinguished people, and worked out this budget which is now $125,500,000 . . . But I am at a loss to understand why [a few weeks earlier] when we were struggling to get the increases not up to $126 million but up to about $112 million, we could get practically no support from the National Institutes of Health. What is the explanation?

Dr. Shannon, who was bearing the brunt of that series of questioning, responded:

> Well, I can give you, to the best of my ability, what I believe is the explanation. It may not be a very satisfactory one . . . I think there is no doubt, in retrospect, that we were in error in estimating our needs.
> Senator Hill: You admit, then, that you were grossly in error?
> Dr. Shannon: Yes, sir.
> Senator Hill: In not supporting this committee's action in increasing these funds. Is that correct?
> Dr. Shannon: In retrospect, those funds could have been well used, yes, sir.
> Senator Hill: They could have been wisely and well used?
> Dr. Shannon: Yes, sir.[43]

In the end, while Congress was impressed that the executive had begun to see the light and was grateful for Secretary Fol-

som's role in the Administration's conversion, it did not consequently fall in line with what was obviously the Administration's—and Secretary Folsom's—plan. For Congress was more
impressed with what it saw as a concession to its own wisdom
over the years than with that wisdom newly found by the Administration.

The Senate Appropriations Subcommittee's report to the
Senate that year, accompanying its proposed appropriations for
the Department of Health, Education and Welfare and the
National Institutes of Health, reviewed past history to justify
present action:

> The Committee has been impressed with the manner in
> which the stimulus of available funds has invigorated the
> entire field of medical research since World War II ended.
> The national capacity for growth in productive medical re-
> search was grossly underestimated, and some of these un-
> derestimates have been made by experts.
>
> A few short weeks after expressing opposition to the com-
> mittee increases [for last year] institute officials proposed,
> and the Department accepted, a budget totaling $126.5
> million, or $14 million in excess of the total budget adopted
> by the Senate.
>
> The committee is of the opinion that the misassessment
> of the situation by the administration last year has been
> repeated this year, and that the proposed budget of $126
> million is therefore inadequate. The committee for this
> reason believes that the action of the House in proposing
> a budget of $135 million is clearly in the right direction.
>
> The lack of foresight and imagination displayed by those
> in the executive branch who are responsible for the grand
> national strategy of medical research has been reflected not
> only in wholly inadequate appropriation requests, but in
> a failure to suggest forms of support realistically adjusted
> to the needs of modern research.[44]

VI   Consolidation: Policies and Politics

It was a grand vision, if not yet a coherent grand strategy, that Congress possessed in 1957. Tutored by experts within and outside government, and especially encouraged by the doctors, scientists, and laymen who made up the medical research lobby, those of the people's elected representatives in positions of relevant responsibility approached the new enlarged national activity eagerly. They were especially attracted to innovation, and their dominant sense of the practical made them in a hurry to see beneficial results of innovation put into widespread application.

In the late 1940's, when the House Appropriations Health Subcommittee had learned during the course of hearings that a new, quicker, surer X-ray technique for the detection of tuberculosis had just been perfected, the committee suggested to the Public Health Service that it send demonstration teams into all the states so that people across the country might benefit from the advance as rapidly as possible. The committee provided a special $3 million for the project, doing so, Representative Fogarty recalled, "without any recommendation from the Bureau of the Budget." [1] When fluoridation came upon the scene, the committee once more urged nationwide demonstrations of the efficacy of the substance, and spontaneously provided money to get the message out to the states. [2] Demonstration teams having subsequently demonstrated their worth, the committee reacted similarly when it learned of a new means of easy, early detection of cervical cancer, and that process was immediately initiated on a wide scale because of swift congressional response. [3]

The congressional approach to medical research, and the application of research and development results, was often like that. A promising new lead, a new finding that needed wider testing to determine its validity, or a new scientist with a new idea excited those members of Congress who were able to do something about the matter, and they often speedily did. Some such possibilities came to their attention in the course of personal meanderings in medical science literature—or medically oriented articles in the Sunday newspapers[4]—prompted by interest, developed simultaneously with developing responsibilities. Often the new possibility was specifically called to congressional attention by members of the medical research lobby or by researchers and administrators at the National Institutes of Health. This could be and often was a most advantageous arrangement.

Unless they themselves were behind the effort to secure congressional interest, hence prompt congressional sponsorship of a new or expanded biomedical research activity, NIH personnel were somewhat nervous about the approach. There was no question that a combination of political power and scientific whimsicality could also produce serious adverse results. And NIH officials were to grow increasingly concerned about what they thought was Mary Lasker's attraction to the "gimmicky." A little biomedical knowledge, they knew, could be a dangerous thing for national biomedical research policy. What they would not admit, even if they perceived it, was that more than a little knowledge about the traditional way NIH proceeded, and knowledge of how to get them to proceed faster or differently, was also dangerous to bureaucratic power.

As in earlier days, when Congress had viewed its proper role as simply that of putting up the money à la Matt Neely and letting the scientists decide what to do with it, congressional health leaders basically relied on the professional judgments of the directors of the component research institutes of NIH as to whether ideas were good, whether new research leads could feasibly be expanded, and how much money could profitably be spent. A favorite Fogarty question to an institute director was: "What would you do with an extra two or three million dollars if the committee and the Congress saw fit to provide it?"[5] In the new era, and the new NIH spirit, most institute directors offered to submit a detailed plan for the use of such extra dollars if they did not have specific ideas right on the spot.

John Fogarty seemed to have a new medical interest every year, often before it became the subject of popular concern. In 1958 he asked the Secretary of HEW, the Surgeon General, and the Director of the National Institute of Mental Health whether anything was being done about the origins of mental retardation.[6] He wanted to know what NIH was doing about multiple sclerosis, Tay-Sachs disease, blindness, cystic fibrosis, retrolental fibroplasia.[7]

The sources of his interests were varied. Some of the specific research ideas he asked NIH witnesses about during hearings were suggested in advance by those officials; or they were suggested by others, "research lobbyists" for example, but subsequently reviewed with institute directors in private before they were explored in the public record. Fogarty, and Hill, knew the importance of "building a record" during the course of hearings on which they could later justify their usual recommended increases in the medical research budget.

A constant source of ideas for both was Mike Gorman, executive director of the National Committee against Mental Illness, organized and co-chaired by Mary Lasker and Florence Mahoney and funded by Mrs. Lasker. Gorman got on well with Fogarty, occasionally feeding him drinks while feeding his ego, and constantly feeding him ideas. Fogarty was less easily flattered than some others. Whatever the original source of his interest in medical research—whether the inspiration of his visionary, nonpartisan predecessor, as Fogarty annually claimed on the floor of the House; his history of heart trouble, as some have suggested; his conversion to the cause by Mrs. Lasker, as some have inferred; or simply the unexpected attainment of a powerful and prestigious chairmanship, with some of the world's most eminent medical statesmen and scholars coming to consult him —it had become a sophisticated, extensive, and genuine interest, and it was not dependent on others' telling him what a great job he was doing for the country and the world. He knew what the bases of his authority were—from the ongoing institutional to the popular and fleeting—and if he thought his role was perhaps a little more important than that of others, he recognized nonetheless that it was a power shared. Others should therefore share the credit.

Mike Gorman had gotten Fogarty and Hill to provide money to start a training program for psychiatrists, under the auspices of the National Institute of Mental Health, in the early fifties. In requesting more funds in 1960 so as to be able to take care of the backlog of approved applications, a perennial justification for increased budgets, Gorman lauded the Congress for having "raised the amount of money available for training from about $6 million in fiscal 1956 to $18 million in 1959." Fogarty was favorable to the idea of an increase, but he responded: "I think you should keep the record straight. It was put in because I think you people were the first to suggest it." [8]

Hearings of the House and Senate Appropriations Subcommittees were structured so as to build a record. But they were not pro forma and not altogether predictable. Nor were chairman Fogarty's perceptions of important research needs always prompted in advance by others. His questions on the subject of problem drinking seemed spontaneous, when Dr. Felix appeared in 1958 to tell the committee what the Mental Health Institute was doing and could do. Their exchange is a vivid illustration of congressional interest leading to a particular research activity.

   Congressman Fogarty: I recall reading that we had between 1.3 million and 2 million problem drinkers in American industry, about 30 cases per thousand workers. That is a pretty high incidence, isn't it?

Dr. Felix: That is; yes.

Fogarty: What are we spending on it?

Felix: . . . Exclusive of what we are spending in our own laboratory, and this is part of our total budget there . . . we are spending $244,278 this year, in 1958, on this problem.

Fogarty: That is just peanuts compared to the problem . . . Don't you think we ought to be doing more?

Felix: Yes, sir; I do . . . [but] there is not enough know-how available among the people who are dealing with alcoholics in the country, aside from a small group, to mount any large scale national program.

Fogarty: If you folks don't make any request of Congress, maybe we ought to take the initiative and tell you to get going. Will that help? . . . I think it is important enough that this committee give some real consideration to giving you some extra funds for this purpose. I would ask you to supply for the record, Dr. Felix, what you would do with $2 million, if this committee granted it, to get started on a real program on alcoholism." [9]

Senator Hill was especially solicitous when unfulfilled research needs or new research activities were suggested by senatorial colleagues. His colleague from Minnesota, Hubert Humphrey, found him most willing to help institute a research program which Humphrey thought was needed. The daughter of a Humphery friend had a condition diagnosed as ulcerative colitis. No one knew much about it, and only three medical scientists, so far as could be ascertained, were working on the problem, one at the Mayo Clinic and two at the University of Chicago Medical School. In the course of his efforts to help his friend, Humphrey found that NIH had no program, and no money, but some interest. It was estimated in 1957 that there might be as many as 500,000 cases of the disease in the United States.[10]

Senator Hill confronted Dr. Shannon with this story; Shannon confirmed the essential facts, and the Senate committee included in its recommended appropriations for the institutes sufficient funds to start a program.

Always the Congress sought scientific confirmation before it plowed ahead. Dr. Shannon later said that Congress never pushed him into research areas he did not want to enter, or forced acceleration of the pace beyond what he thought it should be. The record does not support such a categorical statement, but there is consistent evidence that congressional power was sensitive to the nature of scientific exploration and to the sensibilities of scientists.

In addition to the restraint which congressional leaders imposed upon themselves, there were certain institutionalized restraints which they respected. In the immediate postwar years, with prospects of the boom in sight, NIH officials, especially including the new deputy director, Dr. Cassius J. Van Slyke, had established controls designed to insure high quality research by grantees of the institutes. A system of "study sections" was drafted, under which grant proposals were reviewed for scientific merit and technical feasibility by professional peers of the grant applicant. At the formal direction of the National Advisory Health Council (itself assigned the responsibility to approve all major grants by the Surgeon General), study sections were to pass judgment on proposed projects before they were presented to the advisory councils of each institute for review and recommended action. Indeed, it was precisely these controls on scientific quality of possible research endeavors that encouraged Congress, year after year, to make more money available.

Before he had reassured himself on this score, Congressman Melvin Laird (R., Wis.) who joined the Labor-HEW Appropriations Subcommittee in 1957, suspected there was merit in the charge of some that the Congress was "force-feeding" NIH, providing more money for research than could be soundly used. He raised questions on the point in 1957: "I live around the area of the National Institutes and have talked to people who work out there. They seemed to give me the idea that they were being hard-pressed in finding projects this past year." Replied Dr. Leroy Burney, President Eisenhower's newly appointed Surgeon General: "I am a little surprised at those remarks because, without any stimulation on our part, it soon became known by research institutions outside the National Institutes of Health, that Congress had appropriated more money last year and we received these additional applications . . . So, as I said previously, we were a little surprised that we were able to find as many research groups with the manpower to utilize these funds." [11]

The phenomenon was a continuing one. Surgeon General Burney reported to the House committee in 1960 that despite the heavy increases in funds provided by Congress the previous year, "as in the past, applications that have withstood scrutiny of the scientific community have exceeded in number the number of grants that could be made." [12] In that year, in fact, the criteria for grant approval had been made even stiffer; in signing the 1960 Appropriations Bill, President Eisenhower suggested that in addition to those standards already used, NIH officials and their professional advisers should seek to approve "only those grants which, if not approved, might delay progress in medical discovery, and which, if approved, would not shift essential people away from teaching and medical practice to research.[13] Even so, the volume of approved research projects grew steadily. Chairman Fogarty thought the grants program "must have been pretty good as you were operating before." Naturally Dr. Shannon agreed: "The thing I feel very good about is that the employment of the [new] criteria as rigidly as possible sought the same objectives as we ourselves morally sought. The overall experience has given us a sense of security in our review procedures, that in fact we are doing as good a job as could be done in this type program."[14]

And still there were backlogs in most biomedical scientific fields of research proposals which study sections and advisory councils thought deserving of support if funds were available. The Institute of Arthritic and Metabolic Diseases expected not to be able to fund "about 800 projects that have been approved with high priority by the Council" in 1959.[15] Congress was not moving out blindly or precipitously into unmarked demesnes.

There were other checks and balances, not the least of which was the development of sophisticated knowledge on the part of certain members of Congress, in particular the chairmen and ranking members of the appropriations subcommittees. And they became defter in insuring against anyone's leading them down seductive research paths for other than the right reasons. Mrs. Lasker might push vigorously to get NIH to support a new effort—for example, as happened on a couple of occasions, to support the work of a certain researcher in whose ideas and methods she had become interested. Dr. Shannon and his colleagues might balk, and Mrs. Lasker would then try to get Senator Hill interested in the project. Hill would listen to Shannon's assessment of the value of the proposed project and would usually defer to him.

On the other hand, the congressional research leaders did not automatically adopt new program proposals advanced by the NIH directorate. At one point Dr. Kenneth Endicott, director of the National Cancer Institute, and Dr. Shannon proposed the substantial enlargement of the research program in cancer virology. Apparently their judgment that the time was right for such an effort, a judgment formally if routinely endorsed by the National Advisory Cancer Council, was not sufficient for Senator Hill. For one thing, there was some concern that a new effort in virology might detract from the cancer chemotherapy effort. It became clear that, in this instance, the NIH would have to enlist its own lobbyists if it wished to see its initiative adopted.

At the suggestion of Endicott and Shannon, Hill called Nobel Prize winner Wendell Stanley to discuss the value and the chances for success of the NIH proposal.[16] Stanley was not necessarily the most objective witness that could have been found; he was himself a virology specialist, and he believed that the virological line of investigation held great promise for finding the secret of the persisting mystery of cancer. In fact, it had been Stanley whose earlier work had prompted Endicott's predecessor, Dr. John Heller, to commence a small cancer virology research program in the early 1950's;[17] and the Hill subcommittee had cited Stanley as a major reason for its support of that effort.[18] Thus Hill should not have been surprised that Stanley endorsed the cancer virology project expansion proposed by Endicott and Shannon.

Hill probably was not surprised. But he wanted Stanley's confirmation of the merits before he and his committee colleagues gave the green light to the science bureaucrats. In short, the incident again illustrates the authority of Congress, and particular congressional leaders, in medical research policy and underscores the not imprudent way in which that authority was ordinarily employed.

The congressional procedure did not always produce the decisions he would have preferred, but Dr. Shannon thought it was a sound one. Melvin Laird, in his third year on the subcommittee, still felt occasionally uncomfortable with the influences he and the committee obviously had. Wouldn't it be better, he suggested, if the Congress left more decisions to the institutes? If not, he asked Shannon, "where would you find guidance if you were sitting on this side of the table?" Dr. Shannon replied: "In the first place, I can say that I would not have any one place where I could go because I do not think there is any one person who has the capacity to give sound advice . . . So I do not think we should be the only ones that should advise you how money should be spent; but I think we should be there with your outside advisers in a positive way rather than a negative way, and we cannot be there in a positive way when we have to come up here with a static budget." [19]

The dramatic approach continued to have considerable appeal to the Congress, but medical research sophisticates in the House and Senate, whose numbers gradually increased, came to believe as firmly in the necessity for underpinnings of basic scientific knowledge as did those working in the laboratory. Furthermore, dramatic approaches to problem solving in health were not always eschewed by scientists themselves. In 1957, Laird questioned Surgeon General Burney and Dr. Shannon on the efficacy of the "crash approach" to research. Specifically, he wanted to know if they could provide "any examples of medical research carried out successfully on a crash basis . . . an example of some important discovery that was made by the Federal Government."

Dr. Shannon's experience in discovering and producing an effective antimalarial agent during the war provided him an immediate example. Laird was taken aback:

> Do you have another example?
>
> Dr. Shannon: The use of cortisone and ACTH for arthritis.
>
> Representative Laird: Do you think this is a good method of carrying out research?
>
> Dr. Shannon: No, it is not a good general method . . . One cannot pick a field at random and say we will have a crash effort here. That would be futile.[20]

Yet neither is it a method never to be employed. And by citing cortisone and ACTH as successful examples of crash research Shannon confirmed the wisdom of the ongoing arrangement, for both had been activities spurred vigorously by early congressional enthusiasm.

Representative Taber had asked whether research was not of necessity a long, slow, careful process which could not be speeded up. He was afraid, he said, "we are getting in over our heads and are not going to get as good results as if we were ready to proceed a little more cautiously." The witness, Dr. Harry Weaver of the American Cancer Society, replied: "I know of no single disease, Mr. Taber, that was ever controlled by proceeding cautiously." [21]

Though some thought Congress was proceeding too boldly, it was in fact proceeding cautiously in every way with the possible exception of budget making. The executive budgetary process was one which it had come to view with disenchantment, not to say disdain.

Aside from its own maturing proficiency in recognizing what was and what was not scientifically sound, Congress usually doublechecked its own instincts as regards policy goals and program pace, first with those who had direct responsibility for carrying out or supervising the research activities, then with those whose perspective was from a greater distance but whose judgments were equally professionally sound.

As if to further guard against the possibility of its own whimsicality, Congress suggested ways of insuring that the long view would not be ignored, that the ongoing activities of the institutes would not be upset when new and promising short-term possibilities excited interest and generated special provision of funds. Senator Margaret Chase Smith began in the mid-1950's to urge the National Institutes of Health to develop five-year plans for major research activities.[22] Both appropriations subcommittees took interest in the development of training programs to insure the availability of manpower to undertake research (and for related purposes which at least the sponsors of such programs understood). Basic research became almost as important a consideration to NIH supporters in Congress as to NIH officials. Senator Hill's committee reminded the Senate in 1960 of the balance that must be struck: "Despite the great advances in medicine and its related sciences in recent years man still gropes toward the precise understanding of the causes of many of the major diseases . . . The development of a solid foundation of fundamental knowledge concerning the biological processes is an essential condition for the breakthroughs from which significant victories in major disease areas will flow." [23]

Facilities construction was also a persistent concern; subcommittee leaders almost annually set the stage for executive officials, apparently too timid otherwise, to testify that inadequate facilities were in some instances retarding the pace of research activities, whether in-house on the Bethesda campus or on university campuses and in hospital-medical school complexes.

Senators Hill and Margaret Smith questioned the director of the Neurological Institute, Dr. Pearce Bailey, in 1956:

> Senator Hill: What about your operating facilities there. Do you have sufficient space and room . . . ?
>
> Dr. Bailey: May I answer that by stating that these operations require a terrific amount of electronic equipment. For instance . . .
>
> Senator Smith: Did you say there were sufficient facilities?
>
> Bailey: I have not said yet.
>
> Hill: He has not said yet. He is coming to it. I think he is laying a pretty good predicate.

The predicate laid, the answer comes: Yes, Senator, there is a need.

> Hill: How can we get this room? That is what I want to know. How much money do you want? [24]

Dr. Bailey has really not meant to plead for special additions to his budget, and he is a little nervous about the line of questioning. He defers to his superior: "Dr. Shannon has the answer." Shannon is uncomfortable too. This is the budget that Secretary Folsom has made reasonable for the institutes, and NIH officials are particularly anxious to stay within it. Shannon says the issue of a special facility puts him "in a quandary."

Senator Smith thinks NIH officials should keep their working alliance with Congress and not return to the fickle executive: "Dr. Shannon, do you not think it would be well for some consideration to be given a recommendation that the Congress might consider? These things take time, and it would seem to me that the Congress is the logical place for it to be turned down or promoted. If something is needed to get the full benefit of the money we are spending in research, it would seem that members of Congress would give it serious consideration." [25]

Certainly there was nothing politically incautious about Congressional pushing for increased funds for medical research. A "nonpartisan" foundation for it having been built—a foundation which became more nonpartisanly solid after surviving some partisan assaults—medical research was actively supported from both sides of the aisle.

First of all, the process of socialization among committee members regularly concerned with medical research over the years, a process relating to the subject matter as well as the colleagues involved, has never worked more consistently than here. Most members of the House and Senate Appropriations Subcommittees reviewing medical research activities each year, and many members of the pertinent legislative committees, came to embrace medical research as fervently as any issue in their careers. It was, of course, a safe one: precious few were opposed to it. Yet there are some men in public office who are for or against something not on the basis either of its popularity or its intrinsic worth, but on the basis of how much money it costs; and if it costs too much, they're opposed. On the subject of medical research, to know it was to love it. Or so it seems.

Representative Ben Franklin Jensen (R., Iowa), a fiscal conservative, was a member of the House Appropriations Subcommittee in the 1950's. His most important contribution to legislative deliberations over the years was the regular offering of an amendment to appropriations measures that would cut those appropriations back by 10 percent in every category. But he always exempted the National Institutes of Health. How strongly he felt about the matter is indicated by his colloquy with Dr. Shannon: "I hope, Doctor, that if you need more funds, you will ask for them. This is one place where Jensen is quite liberal. I do not think we should worry about a few million dollars when it comes to finding the cause and cure of these dread human diseases. To do other than what this committee has been doing in furnishing these funds, I think would be almost on the point of criminal." [26]

Senator Robert Byrd (D., W.Va.), who joined the Senate committee in 1957, described the $715 million spent on medical research in the United States from all sources in 1960 as "an infinitesimal amount . . . It is incredible to me that the amount is so small . . . I am pleased to see the House increasing the President's budget . . . and I am wondering if more than that could not be effectively used." [27] Senator Alan Bible (D., Nev.) declared: "It is always a thrilling experience to hear these doctors tell of the advances they are making." [28] Senator Charles Potter (R., Mich.) agreed: "I want to emphasize again how interested I am in this. I know Senator Hill is really a professional in these health programs, but as a lay member of the committee it is always thrilling to me." [29] Representative D. R. (Billy) Matthews (D., Fla.) was a short-term member of the subcommittee but an avid member of the NIH fan club.[30] Even Senator Henry Dvorak (R., Idaho), whose natural and pre-eminent tendency was to save dollars, and whose work on the budget-raising subcommittee made him more than occasionally nervous, sometimes got caught up in the research mystique; he suddenly found himself asking Dr. Felix, one day in 1956, if he believed he was "moving along as rapidly as you can with personnel and with the appropriations to attain the ultimate objective," because he had heard some criticism "of the inadequacy of the program." [31]

Representative Charles Wolverton (R., N.J.), sometime chairman of the House Interstate and Foreign Commerce Committee, praised John Fogarty, saying that he "leaves no doubt that he is the best informed man in Congress on all details affecting our national health program." He continued: "I confess, and in all sincerity frankly state, there has been no service in my many years in Congress that has given me more genuine and real pleasure and satisfaction than that which I have been able to do as a member and chairman at times of the committee in the field of health legislation." [32]

Those members of Congress whose committee contacts with the medical research enterprise had convinced them of its value were not the only ones who spoke up in favor of it whenever the occasion arose. Representative Walter Judd (R., Minn.), a physician, gave the House his slowly developed but certain professional judgment in 1960. At first, he said, back in 1947 when NIH was just getting started in an important way, he had doubted its value and had had reservations about the governments getting into medical research support in such a direct and grandiose fashion. Now he had decided otherwise.

> The National Institutes of Health has no peer anywhere in the world to my knowledge, not only in the magnitude, comprehensiveness, and variety of work being done, but most important of all, as to the superior and scientific excellence of the men and women who have come to work in this excellent institution where the best work in the world is being done on the difficult disease problems that have so far evaded solutions.[33]

Representative Gordon Canfield (R., N.J.) put it more succinctly. He urged his colleagues to visit the NIH campus in Bethesda, saying: "I hope all of you will go out there and see that great human enterprise in action. It is America at its best." [34]

Not everyone was a booster, willing to support medical research at any budgetary level. Some in fact favored cutting back, at least to the level the executive budget makers proposed. Over the years, Congressmen Clarence Cannon and John Taber, alternately chairmen and ranking members of the Appropriations Committee, tried to hold Fogarty and the NIH budget down. "They were much of a kind," commented the *Washington Post* on the occasion of Taber's death; they were "crusty budget cutters, prone to debate money matters at the top of their lungs in rasping voices hard to follow." [35] Sometimes they worked on the matter in the subcommittee; not only did both sometimes show up for the executive session on the NIH appropriation, but in 1956 Taber appointed himself to the subcommittee to see if he couldn't take care of things personally. If he did, it didn't show much in the resulting proposed appropriations. Cannon, his committee colleagues say, did his best to get reductions of the subcommittee members' NIH work in the full committee; but he had little success because Fogarty had the support of a number of other subcommittee chairmen who didn't want their work tampered with by the full committee either. On the floor, Cannon mainly fumed but did not actively try to overturn the health subcommittee's work when the subject came up.

It was not Cannon's preferred style to oppose openly and directly. He could be so charming that he convinced witnesses who appeared before him that he was going to give them everything they had asked for. Mary Lasker came away from a meeting with him once convinced that she had melted his opposition to increases in the medical research budget. She later found out she had misinterpreted his cordiality. Similarly Dr. Howard Rusk, whose mother had been Cannon's schoolteacher in Missouri and who was consequently warmly received by the chairman, learned he had made no headway whatever in convincing Cannon of the need for more dollars; he learned, that is, when the matter went from the personal conversation stage to the stage of voting on the floor of the House.

On the Senate side, Everett Dirksen and Gordon Allott, Republicans, and William Proxmire and Paul Douglas, Democrats, were among those who occasionally tried to hold Senators Hill, Thye, Margaret Smith, Pastore, and Byrd in check. It was never to any avail. Senator Hruska left the subcommittee ostensibly to give a junior colleague a more important subcommittee; but he confesses that a more important reason was that he couldn't do anything "but go along with the increases," and he didn't like that.[36]

The great majority of Congressmen and Senators, however, have supported growing budgets for medical research in the last quarter-century, regardless of what the executive branch has said, and many of them have been outspoken in their support. They would not have consistently done so unless the subcommittees had vividly and comprehensively documented the need and adduced all the proper scientific evidence, and given occasional hints about the possibility of imminent breakthroughs. Perhaps they would not have done so if there had not occasionally been reported a medical advance of real significance. They certainly would not have done so if the people had not themselves thought the medical research enterprise was a good idea, worthy of the full support of all public officials.

Florence Mahoney told every potentially supportive House or Senate member she could about Governor James Cox's readership poll of 1950. To see what kinds of stories his newspapers should feature prominently, Cox polled his many thousand readers, discovering that items on medicine and health had a higher readership than any other category. 92% of readers polled always read health-related news articles. (Only 24 percent usually read editorials.) Representative John Rooney (D., N.Y.), who annually supported John Fogarty's proposed increases in medical research budgets with a speech on the floor of the House, did so in part out of Irish kin. But this man, who made his principal reputation as a budget cutter (whacking away yearly at any excesses he could find in the State Department budget), reminded his colleagues that the Gallup Poll had shown that the public was not only willing to have government spend five times more on cancer research in 1950 than it was spending (80 percent were in favor of increasing the amount); what was more telling, most people (62 percent) would even be willing to pay more taxes to provide for the increased outlays.[37]

Public support was still high in 1962 according to the Senate Democratic Whip, Hubert Humphrey. In an extemporaneous speech giving the "strongest possible endorsement" to the Labor-HEW appropriations subcommittee's effort to increase the NIH budget by an additional $60 million over the House proposal (which in turn was $60 million in excess of the budget estimates), Humphrey reminded the Senate that "every public opinion poll which has ever been conducted on this subject shows this fact: American citizens more heartily approve of this expenditure of their tax funds for support of medical research than for virtually any other research purpose—including space exploration." [38]

It was against this background—of carefully constructed testimony of expert witnesses, of committee member enthusiasm, of general nonpartisan congressional interest, and of wide public appeal—that Congress continued to build a medical research enterprise which was to become accepted as the most important in the history of the world.

As regards the spending levels it sought and achieved, perhaps Congress was not cautious. It did not, in any event, approach medical research and the Institutes of Health in the way that activities and agencies requiring government appropriations are usually approached. The Eisenhower Administration was very much taken aback at Congress' refusal to defer to executive decision making as epitomized in the budgetary process. Secretary Folsom may have been particularly disappointed at the congressional response to his liberal budget proposals for NIH in 1956 and 1957, although in retrospect he was untroubled. If he had any regrets on the matter of the medical research budget and the Administration's inability to gain leadership over it, they were that he was not able to persuade Budget Bureau officials to commitment on a plan for long-range growth such as Senator Smith had proposed. Folsom thought a long-term commitment was not only necessary for the sake of the medical research enterprise, but necessary to demonstrate to genuinely interested, naturally skeptical congressional leaders that the executive shared their sense of importance about the National Institutes of Health and its mission.

Meanwhile, others in the Administration were very unhappy indeed. As a result of Folsom's insistence, the Eisenhower budget for NIH for fiscal year 1957 was $126 million; Congress appropriated $183 million. The next year, the Administration proposed a budget of $190 million; Congress responded by providing the bureau $211 million.

The fiscal 1958 appropriations bill may have been enough to undo Administration planning for NIH. Secretary of the Treasury George Humphrey publicly invited Congress to cut the President's budget. House Republicans responded with special glee, and some of them tried to extend the budget-cutting action to medical research. Charles Wesley Vursell of Illinois, former sheriff of Marion County, said: "I looked into the subject of research. On every page [of the subcommittee report] it was research this and research that. I hope something will be done by amendment or otherwise that will stop some of this research." [39] Even Fogarty's chairman, Clarence Cannon, tried to get "members" to cut the medical research budget: "We cannot meet every need. We cannot support every program. We cannot wipe away every tear." [40] But the Vursell-Cannon effort was utterly hopeless. Though the House slashed away at almost every other budget, that of NIH was not touched.

After 1957 the fiscal liberals within the Administration gave way, and in its struggle with Congress the Administration gave up. For the rest of its life, three fiscal budget periods, it proposed as a budget for NIH precisely the amount Congress had appropriated the previous year. Further, it sought to make stricter the criteria for grant awards, and through the Budget Bureau it doled out medical research money in quarterly allotments, forcing unexpended funds back into the treasury. Congress, thought the executive, was being utterly irresponsible in ignoring the budget process. Further, Budget Director Brundage told Secretary Folsom that spending *that* much money meant buying second-rate research.[41]

To Congress, the most recent Administration tack simply proved executive incapability and disinterest regarding the medical research enterprise. Inflation alone required an annual five-percent budget increase. (By the mid-1960's, 15 percent was the accepted figure.) To move forward required substantially more. It was the Budget Bureau that took the brunt of congressional ire.

The new Secretary of Health, Education and Welfare, Arthur Flemming, urged Chairman Fogarty to consider the "important role that the budget can play and should play in the total field of public administration." [42]

Replied Fogarty: "I appreciate your position. If I were in your position, I would have to take orders too, but sitting on this side of the table, what the Bureau of the Budget does does not make much difference to me. We do not take orders from the Bureau of the Budget. The Congress is responsible for the appropriation of funds." [43]

Senator Hill was in perfect agreement: "The Administration submits budget estimates with reference to funds for health exactly as it submits budget estimates with reference to many different items . . . Then it is a matter for Members of Congress, as direct, chosen representatives of the people, to make a determination as to what funds shall be provided. The Congress, in regard to this bill [providing funds for medical research] is meeting its Constitutional responsibilities." [44]

Melvin Laird, by the 1960's a staunch supporter of the cause, had also become a more willing believer in the nonpartisan approach, especially with a Democratic President in the White

House. Explaining to the House why the committee had once again raised the appropriations for the National Institutes of Health, he offered as a first reason the simple conviction that the activities were "of fundamental importance to the health and well-being of this nation" and as a second that

> the people of this country are fully in support of the com-
> bined effort to enlarge the nation's medical research pro-
> gram . . . I cannot recall that there has ever been a time
> when the action of committee members or of the commit-
> tee itself has been governed by considerations related to
> the party in power. There have been years, however, when
> the executive branch has been unduly restrictive in setting
> the level of its appropriations for medical research activi-
> ties; and this, I am sorry to say, is one of those years.[45]

In the judgment of Congress, the matter had become much more than a question of executive versus legislative responsi-bilities. It had become a question of policy, relating to the na-tional welfare, that should over-ride such considerations as budget-making prerogatives or bureaucratic loyalties. Chair-man Fogarty wanted to know, in 1960, if the National Institute of Mental Health could use more funds for evaluating tranquil-izing drugs for mental patients than the budget estimated. The Director's response illustrates the dilemma of the government official who must serve two masters, especially when they are at odds.

> Institute Director: We have a series of recommendations
> which we can carry through. If more money were available
> it could be wisely spent. However, I want it distinctly un-
> derstood that I am defending the budget in letter and spirit.
> Representative Fogarty: I know that, but I hope I do
> not have to repeat too often that when I ask you a specific
> question I want you to give us an answer as far as your
> professional judgment is concerned . . . regardless of the

limitations that you are under as far as the Department or the Bureau of the Budget is concerned. Is that plain, Doctor?

Institute Director: Yes, sir. It is my professional opinion, sir, that this program could be expanded beyond the $2 million level if it is the wish of Congress that we do so.[46]

It was, to be sure, the wish of Congress that the program be expanded.

If not very restrained in their budgetary approach to medical research, the House and Senate committees were not completely without balance. Senator Chavez emphasized to his colleagues how much money was going for war and defense: "I am now chairman of the subcommittee that handles the $41 million destruction bill, the Department of Defense appropriations bill. I note there is requested an increase of $209 million to this bill for medical research . . . Yesterday we had hearings [on] a request . . . for restoration of $290 million for an aircraft carrier, a conventional one." [47]

Representative George Miller (D., Cal.), chairman of the Science and Astronautics Committee, urged the House to go along with the Labor-HEW Appropriations Subcommittee's proposed increases for medical research, reminding his colleagues of the recently enacted $300 million appropriation for development of new missiles: "An economy that can stand that expenditure can afford additional expenditures for health." Besides, Representative J. Vaughan Gary (D., Va.) told the House, not only is health research a good and worthy cause, but the Subcommittee he chaired would see to it that the House appropriated less than the President's total budget recommended; he was planning to bring to the floor of the House a much reduced foreign aid bill.[48]

The fiscal prudence of Congress' approach to medical research may nonetheless be debated. Congressional boldness in seizing and pre-empting an important policy area is unquestionable.

And congressional occupation of the premises became, with time, an increasingly enlightened one. "In essence," reported the Senate Appropriations Committee to the Senate in 1960, "though it has not been so stated, there has come into being a national policy that calls for a sustained and expanded research attack against disease . . . The Nation cannot afford to do other than to provide adequately for the support of trained scientists. To pursue any other course of action would be specious economy and at the same time a rejection of the great humanitarian principles for which our Nation stands. For our people are one of our primary natural resources. The health is related to their productivity and to the strength and well being of our country." [49]

To achieve the ultimate policy goal of conquering disease and improving and extending the people's health, the biomedical scientific enterprise must be built up and institutions and individual researchers supported. That would take great amounts of money, and Congress was willing, even determined, to spend whatever it might take to move the enterprise to optimum productivity as quickly as possible. His colleagues would not necessarily go all the way with John Fogarty in his vow to make sure every competent investigator had as much money as he needed; but they agreed with his aims.

Further, the legislative branch was no longer willing simply to put up the money. Even in its most formal, fiscal action vis-à-vis NIH—the provision of appropriations—Congress, through its two committees, exerted influence on substance, quality, size, and pace. The Labor-HEW appropriation bill, said John Fogarty's Democratic colleague from Missouri, Leonore Sullivan,

> is a most remarkable piece of legislation . . . It uses the vehicle of an appropriation bill to do much more than merely provide funds for some Government agencies. As usual, the report accompanying the bill prods, stimulates, encourages, directs and scolds the agencies having such tre-

mendous responsibility for the health and well-being of the American people to do a better job with the generous funds we give them—and to use more imagination and courage in pressing new avenues of service to the public.[50]

The legislative approach to medical research policy, then, was not, despite superficial appearances, just an automatic liberal fiscal one. It reflected substantive knowledge, certainty of goals, and sophistication regarding means. Whereas the executive took an old-fashioned, steady if not static, incremental budgetary approach, Congress evidenced flexibility. It thought large, providing for the long-run and for the supplementary and the complementary as well as for the direct, the dramatic, the immediately appealing. It acceded to the felt need of researchers and research administrators while continuing to scout for new possibilities. Where the odds were reasonable, it pushed the normally conservative research enterprise faster than it might go if left to its own ways. More sophisticated congressional policy makers knew that medical research was sustaining medical school budgets and some university science departments. On the whole the approach was balanced as well as bold.

Increasingly confident of its role, and increasingly convinced that the executive did not intend to offer leadership, Congress all but ignored the traditional executive policy-directing, pace-setting machinery. The Surgeon General of the Public Health Service was a decreasingly important figure. So was the Secretary of Health, Education and Welfare, except when periodically called upon to arbitrate major or minor disputes. The Budget Bureau, smug and pietistic about what it thought should be its exclusive role as national policy coordinator, unwilling or unable to keep up either with scientific or political trends, effectively dealt itself out of the game. In the area of medical research support, it was not only ignored but scorned by Congress.

Congress was not, of course, the only locus of decisions on policy. The National Institutes of Health developed not a little power in the late fifties and early sixties. And the medical research lobby was just reaching its peak of activity and perceived influence. Further, the power Congress had developed was not located in one place or one man; and there were still, within and without the legislature, some known critics of both congressional power and everexpanding medical research activities. Congress, however, was now at the center, the acme of this one policy process. Fully understanding the importance of its mission, fully convinced of the importance of its goals, it proceeded intelligently and logically to lay out a plan for their attainment.

Pure logic, of course, was not the only means employed in building support for its purposeful plans. Senator Hill knew that emotion also had its place in the scheme of things. As he opened the annual hearings on appropriations for the National Institutes of Health for 1960, he thought it was appropriate, he said to his colleagues,

> that we take notice of the passing of our former Secretary of State, John Foster Dulles, who rose indomitable from many a crisis, only to fall victim to the most dreaded killer of our time, cancer.
>
> Cancer, that most ancient and accursed scourge of mankind, has over the past few years robbed the United States Senate of some of its greatest leaders: Robert A. Taft, Arthur Vandenberg, Kenneth Wherry, Brien McMahon, and Matthew Neely.
>
> What more fitting, more meaningful, or more reverent memorial could there be than a high resolve on the part of those assembled here and elsewhere throughout this great land to redouble our efforts against the monstrous killer which struck Mr. Dulles down and which will claim the lives of 250,000 more Americans before this year has ended? [51]

VII Lobbying Medical Professionals and Professional Medical Lobbyists

Government's grand entrance into medical research after World War II was no more potent than the bold entry of laymen into the health domain, once considered acreage exclusively to be tended and tilled by professional medical men. Of course, the two events were related.

The consequences are still flowing from the takeover of the American Society for the Control of Cancer by the Laskers and their friends Elmer Bobst, James S. Adams, Eric Johnston, and Emerson Foote.

The director of the Society at the time, Dr. Clarence Cook Little, represented to the new lay directors the embodiment of the problem: medical practitioners and medical scientists were overly cautious; they thought small; they were primarily protective of their professional positions; and they were especially distrustful of the federal government. In particular, the medical directors of disease-oriented societies were apprehensive, in these early days, that the federal government's enlarged involvement in medical research would push them off to the sidelines, causing private funds and the interest of private citizens to wane. The streamlined American Cancer Society not only raised more money than its predecessor organization had thought possible; it also laid to rest the fear of waning funds and interest. What the government's expanded cancer research efforts actually demonstrated was that enlarged governmental efforts spurred private interest. As federal money for the National Cancer Institute went up year after year, so private contributions to the Cancer Society increased. (In 1970 the American Cancer Society raised $70 million.)

The lesson was an important one. It was no doubt instrumental in producing a new posture among private organizations concerned with particular diseases; it also contributed to the rise of additional organizations. As federal money for medical research increased, and as new categorical institutes were established by the Public Health Service, new associations and societies with particular health aims that often paralleled those of the research institutes came into being. Some preceded the institutes, of course, and some continued to operate in seeming unconcern about what the government was doing in their area of special medical interest. Some had more narrowly focused interests than the research institutes. But all of those organizations which followed the lead of the American Cancer Society —pleading for new or expanded government research activity in their areas of interest, in the fearless knowledge that their own organizational well-being would not be infringed upon and might be enhanced—served the cause well.

The second step of the laymen was equally portentous. When Leonard Scheele agreed to include a provision for lay membership on the National Advisory Council within the Heart Institute Act of 1948, and subsequently got it extended to all advisory councils, he subjected his fellow medical professionals to a persistent prodding they were very much unaccustomed to. For one thing, the lay members first and most frequently appointed were Mrs. Lasker and Mrs. Mahoney; other spirited lay appointments from time to time included Mike Gorman and Mrs. Lasker's sister, Mrs. Almon Fordyce.

A scientist member recalled that at an early meeting of the National Advisory Council there was a prolonged discussion over whether to approve an item in a grant proposal for a small research instrument. A lay member spoke up: "Gentlemen, I thought you were interested in this work. [If so] you've got to spend millions, not hundreds." [1] Maurice Goldblatt, whom Scheele appointed to the Cancer Council, whose fortune was made in a chain of department stores in Chicago that he had founded and whose most passionate concern was conquering disease which had from time to time afflicted himself and his family, wanted his Council colleagues to approve every project that held out the faintest glimmer of hope of discovery. Dr. Scheele says Goldblatt would listen to medical professionals debate research techniques and institutional settings and especially budget figures, and would finally explode: "We are talking about life and death. How can you worry about money?" [2] Dr. Scheele summed up the impact of the laymen on the councils after the first couple of years: "The enthusiasm of the lay members is very hard to keep up with. We medical people are very conservative. These people constantly stimulate us and remind us of our responsibilities." [3]

General David Sarnoff, chairman of the Radio Corporation of America, said that the advantage laymen brought to the medical research field was the same that had been ascribed to him by one of his company's scientists, whom he had asked to develop an air-conditioning unit which had no moving parts, was noiseless, and was simple to operate. The reply was: "Boss, it is wonderful to have an imagination like yours unrestricted by the slightest knowledge of the facts." [4]

If such a thing were possible, the Laskers would just as soon have seen the medical research enterprise operate without doctors. Most doctors, they thought, were possessed of a "small business mentality." The little store of facts they held restricted their vision and imagination. For Albert Lasker, cancer research, like any other enterprise, had to be big if big results were to be expected. There seemed to be no question in his or his cohorts' minds that once a sufficient research effort was mounted—however big it might be—cancer could be conquered.

First, of course, you had to organize, perhaps even institutionalize. The Laskers had already established the Lasker Foundation in New York during the war. Its annual awards to pioneering medical scientists and, subsequently, to public officials who had made significant contributions to medical research

(Lister Hill and John Fogarty were among the first recipients) and to journalists writing on medical subjects helped generate an atmosphere conducive to the expansion of research activities and funds. The Foundation financed the National Health Education Committee, Inc., which produced figures on deaths, disabilities, and income losses accountable to disease and illness—statistics which were widely used by *and on* public officials and others in positions of influence, in pursuit of greater funds.[5] What was now needed, in addition, was someone in Washington watching over the medical research scene full-time, scouting for potential allies, reinforcing existing support, keeping present friends happy, and, especially, coordinating the annual approach to Congress for greater outlays for the Cause.

One layman who had proven himself a versatile and effective promoter of health causes was Mike Gorman. He had been "discovered" by Florence Mahoney, who was impressed with his 1940's journalistic crusade against conditions in the state mental institutions in Oklahoma. She got her husband to bring Gorman to Miami to do the same thing in Florida. His series of articles for the *Miami Daily News* was equally dramatic and equally successful. Reinforced by a bit of focused on-the-scene lobbying in Tallahassee, the result of the "exposé" was an appropriation of $6 million for mental health programs from the Florida legislature.[6]

From there, Mrs. Mahoney pointed Gorman in the direction of Washington, where he became Executive Director of the President's Commission on the Health Needs of the Nation, chaired by Dr. Paul Magnuson. The Commission's report, written by Gorman, built a careful case for considerably expanded federal efforts in medical research. When the job *for* the government was done, that left the job to be done *on* the government. Mary Lasker and Florence Mahoney thought nobody could do it better than Mike Gorman.

The result was the creation of the National Committee on Mental Health, subsequently changed to the National Committee Against Mental Illness. The chairman of the Committee, set up in 1953, was Mrs. Lasker. Other members included Governors Earl Warren of California, Luther Youngdahl of Minnesota, Sid McMath of Arkansas, and Dan Thornton of Colorado; also Congressman Keefe, Elmo Roper, the poll-taker, and Mrs. Lasker's sister, Mrs. Fordyce.[7] Despite its delimited title, reflecting Mike Gorman's keenest health interest, the job was to look after the whole waterfront, and Gorman did so with relish. Mrs. Lasker funded the operation.

By the mid-1960's Gorman could report that he was "on a first-name basis" with 150 to 175 members of the House of Representatives.[8] He could also call up a few Senators with no trouble. More than occasionally, Senators and Congressmen called him. For one thing, they wanted him to be sure to produce some expert witnesses, by which they meant witnesses who were both expert in their professional medical fields and expert at being witnesses. From 1953 until the present day, Gorman has been glad to oblige. He has set a pretty good example himself, displaying to the House and Senate subcommittees a knowledge of recent relevant statistics, a burning concern for the victims of mental illness and of cancer (of which his wife died), and a dramatic verbal flair that almost makes up for the one deficiency he and his lay colleagues all have in the eyes of Congress: lack of a science or medical degree.

Not that the committees only hear and are influenced by medical practitioners or medical scientists. Lay witnesses are very important, for among other things congressional sponsors of medical research want to show is that the Cause generally, and increased appropriations for it specifically, have support from every quarter of the citizenry.

Lister Hill said that in deciding how much money to get the Senate to provide for medical research and where to get the National Institutes of Health to spend it—his dual job over the years—the "citizen" and "outside professional" witnesses who testified annually before his subcommittee were a greater help than any other source. "They had the knowledge, the expertise, the facts." [9]

If they had dramatic appeal as well, so much the better. Senator Chavez called as a witness one year author John Gunther, who had just lost his son from a particularly virulent form of cancer and whose book about the terrible experience, *Death Be Not Proud*, had reached wide audiences through edited versions appearing in the *Reader's Digest* and the *Ladies Home Journal*.[10] John Fogarty brought Daniel McIver of Rhode Island, a victim of multiple sclerosis, to testify on the inadequacy of the research program in that field in 1956. His testimony, dramatized by his condition, moved the committee members. "I know I will not say anything embarrassing to you," said Congressman Thomas Hand (R., N.J.), "when I say how deeply I feel for the courage with which you have adjusted to this situation." [11]

Members of Congress with personal knowledge of dread diseases also made good witnesses. Senator Charles Tobey of New Hampshire pleaded with the Senate committee in 1949 to add $200 thousand to the NIH budget so that a program of studies in cerebral palsy—from which his daughter had just died—and in multiple sclerosis and epilepsy could be begun.[12] Senator Richard Neuberger (D., Ore.), fighting for his life against cancer, appeared yearly before the Senate committee until his death in 1960 to urge generous appropriations for cancer research.[13]

Chairman Fogarty of the appropriations subcommittee explained to the House in 1952 that "when we hold these hearings on the Public Health Service we have the head of every institute . . . and at the conclusion we invite some of the outstanding physicians of the country to come and give their views as to how these research grants are working and the advances that are being made . . . and whether they think we are getting results from the expenditure of Federal monies for research into these leading causes of death." [14]

That year the committee had heard, in addition to prominent

individual medical doctors and medical scientists, the paid executives or other representatives of the American Cancer Society, National Mental Health Committee, American Heart Association, Muscular Dystrophy Association, Cerebral Palsy Association, and Multiple Sclerosis Society. Each of them, of course, wanted Congress to appropriate additional funds for the research institute supporting work in the medical area of its interest. Others were added, or added themselves, to the list of annual supporters of increased medical research funds: the Rheumatism Foundation; the National Committee for Research in Neurological Disorders; Research in Schizophrenia Endowment, Inc.; Research to Prevent Blindness, Inc.; National Cystic Fibrosis Association.

Some of them seem to have been set up at the suggestion of members of Congress. In 1953 in an exchange with Dr. Pearce Bailey, director of the National Institute of Neurological Diseases and Blindness, Fogarty asked whether there was any outside "coordinating committee" on progress in neurology. At the hearings the following year Bailey reported that there were two new organizations particularly interested in the work of his institute, the National Committee for Research in Neurological Diseases and the National Committee for Blinding Eye Diseases and Disability.[15]

Sometimes those institutes with no supportive "professional associations" or "citizen witnesses" were left out when second helpings of dollars were served up by the committees. The Institute of Allergy and Infectious Diseases and the Institute of General Medical Sciences sometimes even found their budgets cut; other years Fogarty and Laird, or Hill and his ranking opposite, seemed to take pity on them and gave them a little extra because nobody else was there to speak up for them.

As John Fogarty's explanation to the House in 1952 suggests, it was mainly the doctors, the medical professionals, whose testimony year after year was principally relied upon to persuade parent appropriations committees and parent legislative bodies that more money was needed and could be used to the advantage of science and the ultimate health of the nation. Special witnesses like John Gunther may have moved subcommittee members to greater compassion and, more important, greater solidarity, but hard-nosed appropriations committee members were more impressed with expertise, scientific assessments, professionalism than with emotional pleas—or at least they pretended to be.

Congressman H. R. Gross (R., Iowa) was particularly concerned to hear the chairman of the House Appropriations Subcommittee suggest that, beyond the increases for medical research in the regular annual budget, there would be a supplemental appropriation request which might include still more funds for NIH. Could the subcommittee not hold the figures down, he asked. No, replied Fogarty, nor should they necessarily try to do so: "This bill is going to grow and grow and grow and grow and grow, and I think it should." But, asked Gross, "What progress has been made in heart research and cancer research and its application for the enormous amount of money that has been spent for research in this field?" [16]

Fogarty replied: "I am not a physician, as the gentlemen know. We do have physicians in the House. In addition, we have listened to hundreds of them in the past 10 or 15 years, some of them the very best in the world . . . They tell us that because of the advances in heart surgery over the last 4 or 5 years untold thousands of people are walking around today who otherwise could not have survived their heart ailments." [17] The counsel of "some of the best doctors in the world" was apparently sufficient for Mr. Gross. There were no more questions.

Further, it was not just that the learned doctors knew their professional fields better than almost anyone else. They had "the facts" in another sense. More often than not they served as members of the advisory councils of the component institutes of NIH; hence each knew what his institute had originally proposed as a budget and what plans there were for the future, if, that is, the money were sufficient and the executive budg-etary-program coordination system permitted the implementa-tion of those plans.

Such witnesses as Dr. Paul Dudley White posed a triple threat to congressional penny-pinchers. He was one of the most emi-nent heart specialists in the country, having treated a range of important persons from President Eisenhower to Congressman Fogarty. He was a member (or former member, depending on the year) of the National Advisory Heart Council, which re-viewed potential heart research projects for the National Heart Institute and regularly reviewed as well the state of the art of heart research, new ideas and imminent breakthroughs, and proposed budgets to take advantage of all of those. Yet he repre-sented a nongovernmental, outside, "objective" assessment of a citizens' association whose concern was simply the eradica-tion of heart disease, the health of fellow citizens.

Dr. White officially spoke for a citizens committee for heart research. Explaining to Senator Stennis what the "citizens com-mittee" was, White said that although it was totally separate from the National Advisory Heart Council, the Council "has backed them unanimously." In essence, the purpose of the citi-zens committee was "to put these acts [creating categorical dis-ease research institutes] into effect." [18]

Dr. Sidney Farber was even more precise in explaining to the House subcommittee the nature and the purpose of the citizens committee on cancer research.

> Farber: The budget which I am about to present grew out of the studies of a number of informed individuals who are deeply interested in the cancer program in this country. Their deliberations were finally put into form for presenta-tion before this committee in a special meeting held last night by a group of citizens. These people are all present or past members of the National Advisory Cancer Council.

It is their unanimous recommendation which I propose to present to you, Mr. Chairman.

Chairman Fogarty: Has the Advisory Council concurred?

Dr. Farber: They have been asked not to give advice as a council. So they are giving this advice as private citizens.[19]

Inasmuch as the advisory councils were restrained from lobbying, "citizens committees" were created to fill that role.

There was one more reason the citizens committee representatives felt justified in perennially asking for more: they had "updated" information. The institute budgets, like all other federal agency budgets, are drawn up many weeks before being reviewed and finally approved by the Bureau of the Budget and often many months before they are considered by the congressional appropriations committees. If the research enterprise is to any degree one with internal dynamics, rather than a predictably maneuvered activity, it can be imagined that "needs" might in fact change. Dr. Shannon suggested as much in replying to a puzzled Congressman Laird about why he, Shannon, didn't mind if the House subcommittee changed the figures NIH had specified it needed; it was not that anything was wrong with medical research management as Laird had suggested, but that "something is wrong with the mechanics of budget making." [20]

The time lag between budget composition and congressional consideration, underscored by recent deliberations of the various advisory councils, gave the congressional subcommittees substantial reason, they felt, to rely more heavily on other guidelines than the executive budget recommendations for the National Institutes of Health. It seemed a reasonable position. To paraphrase Dr. Johnson, what is striking about this system of securing more funds for whatever cause is not that it is done, but that it is not done more frequently. Rarely if ever has any government agency or government-sponsored activity been so consistently supported by such a strong network of friends operating in such a systematic way.

Dr. Farber offered a simple explanation of why he wanted the Senate to approve $5 million more for cancer research than the President's budget had asked: "The President's budget was prepared at a time by men who did not have available the figures that I have been giving you [on the number and cost of approved research projects] and this explains in great part the disparity between the two figures." [21] Another citizen-witness doctor reported to the Senate Committee: "I have been informed recently by a member of the Council, which information I am sure I am permitted to pass on to you, that following the last meeting just a few weeks ago there was approximately $700,000 in approved research grants that could not be paid because of insufficient funds. Even more startling is the fact that there were more than $3,100,000 in new grants that could not be acted upon for the same reason." [22]

Various administration officials, at the time and later, thought the citizen witnesses padded their figures as a calculated move in the sequence of presentations-deliberations-decisions. There was no doubt about the pattern: NIH or HEW cut the original separate institute budgets and the Bureau of the Budget cut the resulting figure. The House then added funds, next the Senate increased them—both actions based largely on the testimony of the outside professionals—and the final compromise was somewhere between the House and Senate figures. The "citizen budgets" were always inflated, says a former Assistant Secretary of HEW. Moreover, they were irresponsible, adds a former Surgeon General. Not so, reports one doctor: The process used by citizens committees is like all others; figures are proposed by various individuals, and in the end the estimates of what can be effectively spent are a compromise between the high figures and the low figures.

Dr. Shannon would not comment on the accuracy of "citizens committee" budgets, but in 1965 he reflected that on the whole the citizens groups had been more helpful and progressive than some of the directors of the institutes.[23]

The system of providing, direct to Congress, expert, professional, recent, relevant advice, based in part on inside information but delivered with outside objectivity, was practically impervious. Medical doctors and scientists persuaded congressmen on the basis of supposedly firm dollars-and-cents estimates, and on the basis of scientific prognostications of advancement or of rapid deterioration and retrogression if funds weren't supplied. They had just about everything going for them, including perceived popular support and a subcommittee audience ready to believe. Even so it took some doing to get the right witnesses.

The first test was that the doctor-scientist be capable of painting a broad picture but filling in details on request. The second was that he use language that simultaneously demonstrated his scientific proficiency and an interest in communicating with ordinary mortals. Usually, says Mike Gorman, the language of physicians and medical researchers is "extremely technical, jargonistic." He continues: "I *forbid* doctors to use the term 'myocardial infarction,' I say, 'You call it heart attack or you leave the room.' That and 'no smoking.' Those are the two rules. It's hard to find the right combination."[24]

The right combination, then, is professional excellence (elder statesmen or younger pace-setters are the most impressive), inside information (members or former members of advisory councils), plain English, and evidence of passionate conviction. The roster of professional witnesses has changed very little through the years. Gorman gives a clue to the reason: "DeBakey is unique; he has the aura of the surgeon, he's articulate, enthusiastic. Most doctors are not enthusiastic, not used to the verbal give and take. The Rusks, Farbers, DeBakeys have evangelistic pizzazz. Put a tambourine in their hands and they go to work."[25]

It doesn't hurt, of course, if a professional witness is from the same state as a key member of the committee. When the reluctant Roman Hruska of Nebraska was on the Senate Committee in 1960, one of the witnesses was Dr. Cecil Wittson, chairman of the Department of Neurology and Psychiatry at the University of Nebraska School of Medicine. No doubt his testimony made it harder than ever for Hruska not "to go along." Said Dr. Wittson: "We are not doing everything that is reasonably possible to meet the needs for personnel, or to develop new methods of treatment, or uncover the causes of diseases." [26]

The subcommittees know what they need, know what they must emphasize each year in order to get their already established design past the hierarchical review system. Some years they want the accent placed more on the fiscal side, and they exact specific statements from the doctor-witness: "I can assure you that [the figure we suggest] is a figure based upon scrutiny of the presently available funds and familiarity with the program of cardiovascular disease." [27] Other years the emphasis must be on progress made to date. John Fogarty pressed Dr. Paul Dudley White on this aspect from time to time:

> Every year we have attempted to keep up somewhere near the approved applications on research that have come out of your Advisory Council . . . You mentioned 3 or 4 areas where we have made definite advances in cardiovascular diseases. So there isn't any question in your mind that this money is being well spent, that we are advancing and getting greater knowledge every year because of the amount of money we are spending on research; is that a fair statement?

Dr. White replied: "May I say that the difference in the situation when I was a medical student 40 years ago . . . and now, in the whole field of medicine and in cardiovascular disease in particular is the difference in night and day. We were really in the dark ages of medicine then. The dawn is here. I don't think we are quite fully in the golden age of medicine but we are getting there." [28]

White's response is close to the ideal for ordinary purposes and in ordinary times: the layman, including the congressman, perceives evidence of real progress and money well spent; the doctor-scientist has not had to strain to single out government-sponsored research for specific credits on specific disease advances; and there is vision and passion in the physician's professional judgment. But it may not be enough, especially if the subcommittee chairman and his allies expect trouble "upstairs."

On other occasions Fogarty had asked White to spell out the progress and promise, and particularly the projected use of additional dollars, in finer point. "We need more details to provide answers to questions on the floor . . . if we had that spelled out project by project, I think you would make a much stronger case. It would be easier for us to explain it upstairs." [29]

It was the requirement of drama and passion that was particularly hard for some of the doctor witnesses, at least in their early appearances. Dr. Isadore Ravdin was coached in the art of testifying by Chairman Fogarty in 1958:

> Fogarty: This budget that the President has given us is going backward and not ahead . . . What does that mean so far as the general public is concerned?
>
> Ravdin: It means a great impediment to progress in the field of cancer.
>
> Fogarty: I thought it was worse than that.
>
> Ravdin: I would personally consider it catastrophic.[30]

That was more like it.

Similarly, Senator Hill coached another professional medical scientist who was a novice as a witness:

> Hill: I have long felt that we have not done what we should in this area . . . Do you have enough people now who can go forward if you have the funds?
>
> Witness: We do not have the full number of people we need.

Hill: In other words, your plea today then would be for the funds to train the people who can do this job?

Witness: Correct.

Hill: Something that we have been woefully lacking in the past. Is that not right?

Witness: That is correct.

Hill: . . . We have really done so little in this field. So little in this field.

Witness [finally getting warmer]: The situation in the hearing field insofar as trained investigators and trained teachers is acute.

Hill [pleased]: That is right, compelling, is it not?

Witness: That is correct.

Hill: Compelling.[31]

When a witness had done a particularly good job, Senator Hill was particularly pleased and responded with an extra dose of his usual graciousness: "This has been a magnificent presentation. You have been a wonderful team here today. You have done a beautiful job and have been so helpful. You have made so many fine contributions. You have been so informative, so interesting and so challenging. We certainly want to thank you and express our deep appreciation." [32]

A very good professional witness, in both senses of the word, was Dr. Cornelius Traeger, medical director of the Multiple Sclerosis Society and a director of the Arthritis and Rheumatism Foundation. He was daring in approach, direct in language. Was there a need for new facilities? "I'm glad you asked that question. The answer is yes without qualification [and not to do it] would be a disaster." [33] What about the suggestion that expanding research efforts in a given categorical disease field might adversely affect the total medical manpower supply and draw physicians from practice into the laboratory? "Statistical nonsense!" Dr. Traeger warned, superfluously in view of his record, that he was going to speak bluntly. Go right ahead, replied Senator Hill; "we know you shoot better when you shoot from the hip." [34]

It was that certain lack of caution that separated the good witnesses from the lackluster ones, who might nonetheless be good professionals. Sometimes when the old pros needed a break or an assist from the annual dog-and-pony performance before the subcommittees, substitutes were sent or help brought. One year Dr. Farber brought Dr. Charles Huggins of the University of Chicago Medical School, a Lasker Award winner. To Dr. Farber's great chagrin, and Mike Gorman's ire, Dr. Huggins said in response to a question by a committee member that he agreed that there ought to be some ceiling on research funds; otherwise, he volunteered, they could be wasted. He personally thought that federal medical research budgets had been progressing at about the right speed.[35] That spontaneous judgment would have shaken the medical research lobby at any point in time over the last quarter of a century. It came in 1955, and the only reason it didn't cause more ripples then was that, at that stage, few eyes were focused on the medical research enterprise and fewer on the research lobby. If they had been so focused, Dr. Huggins might have seriously retarded the Cause.

There were probably others that shared that view. Indeed, it was probably the typical view among medical scientists—precisely the problem, as the medical research lobbyists saw it. But it was not a "helpful" point of view, as Senator Hill might put it; there was no point in the committees listening to such testimony as that. Of course the witnesses whom the subcommittee heard were all distinguished, learned men, replied Senator Gordon Allott (R., Colo.) to a new zealous friend of the Cause, Senator John O. Pastore; but the distinguished Senator from Rhode Island would have to admit that they were all "from the same side of the slate." [36]

As it was, Dr. Huggins' testimony was quickly challenged by Dr. Charles Cameron, himself an old pro who no doubt had had to pass the Lasker salesmanship test before he got his job as Medical and Scientific Director of the American Cancer Society. In fact, said Dr. Cameron, the Cancer Institute budget was very conservative; it certainly was not sufficient in terms of manpower training funds. "I think," he continued, "that if Congress were to flood the Institute with money it would simply mean cancer research would get down into institutions which are not now receiving money . . . it would mean providing a base for the development of men who are going to carry on the best research." [37]

It was the medical men who delivered the message—whose diagnosis and prognosis were the most persuasive, whether most reassuring or most alarming. The logistics, including the selection of physicians and scientists, and often their education and training, were managed by the lay professionals. And they were the ones who suggested calling a doctor in the first place.

In 1960 President Eisenhower—very possibly genuinely fed up with the Congress for continuing to ignore his budget recommendations, especially as regards the Department of Health, Education and Welfare, and in any case realizing that congressional spending could be a vote-getting issue in the upcoming elections—let it be known that he might veto the Labor-HEW appropriations bill for fiscal year 1961. For NIH alone, the Congress had appropriated $547 million, $147 million more than the President had asked. A veto message had already been prepared by the Undersecretary of HEW, Elliot Richardson.[38] The medical research lobby had no direct access to the White House. In fact, with Secretary Folsom's departure, they had few high-level friends left in the executive branch. Mary Lasker, however, is as ingenious as she is indefatigable. The plan she developed was as follows: her good friend Jules Stein, head of the Music Corporation of America, had a good friend who in turn was a frequent golf partner of the President and, happily, was scheduled to play golf with the President in Newport. His favor to his friend Stein was to convince the President of the alarming consequences for the health of the nation if funds for medical research were reduced by reason of a presidential veto. Stein and Farber flew to Newport. Farber did most of the talking, summing up his picture of possible advances or potential horrors (depending on the President's actions) with the observation that the Allies' success—and General Eisenhower's—in the Normandy invasion was the result of his having been provided every weapon and every other resource he might need to do the job. The President, says Dr. Farber, seemed pointedly impressed. He directed an aide to call Secretary Flemming and make an appointment with him for Dr. Farber. Dr. Farber was authorized to tell the Secretary that the President backed him and his associates on the NIH budget. In the end there was no veto.[39]

To gradually build support ahead of time is better than to have to connive and scurry to prevent last-minute problems. And the more support you have built, the more congressional friends you have, the harder it is for the executive to do anything to retard the Cause. Ideally, of course, you have good, important friends in both places. In 1967, Mike Gorman persuaded Senate Majority Leader Mike Mansfield of Montana to host a luncheon for a number of his colleagues so that they could be brought up to date on the latest advances, and projected needs, in the field of heart research. Thirty-six Senators attended, and heard Dr. Michael DeBakey, the heart surgery and heart transplant pioneer, and other distinguished cardiologists describe the state of heart medicine. The doctors also reminded the Senators that one million of their fellow citizens die of heart disease each year. Gorman saw to it that the meal was edible and that "the tables were bussed properly." Senator Mansfield made opening, sympathetic remarks. Mrs. Lasker paid the check.[40]

It should be stressed that the medical professionals whom the lay lobbyists seem to "manage," producing the right one in the right setting at the right time, are no puppets. They are stars, and when they appear for an important performance it is not simply because their managers have ordered them to do so. They are true believers. And they believe that their role in convincing members of Congress, an occasional President, and portions of the public about the need to advance the cause of health through increased medical research efforts has been a central one.

As in any good production with a series of convincing performances, it is difficult to imagine the play without any of the principal and supporting characters. But the degree of importance of any given role may be differently judged by the player and his fellows.

Colonel Luke Quinn, an old friend of John Fogarty's, joined the medical research lobby when he retired from the Air Force in 1952. Fogarty got his friend interested in the Cause, got the American Cancer Society to retain him, and got Mrs. Lasker to increase her contribution to the Society. Quinn had known a good many congressmen from his days in the Legislative Liaison Office of the Air Force, and he liked the Hill with its inside politicking. Quinn, in fact, saw medical research mainly as a political proposition. For one thing, although Fogarty and Hill both developed deep, genuine interest in the scientific intricacies of research and the application of research results to the people's maladies, and although they held each other in real respect, they did not communicate directly. That could be a problem in the development of any empire. One of Quinn's, and Gorman's, functions was to see to it that the chairmen of the House and Senate subcommittees each knew what the other was thinking and planning.[41]

According to Quinn and others, the testimony of eminent physicians and scientists like Farber, DeBakey, Ravdin, Traeger, Rusk, Rhoads, et al., made little personal difference to Fogarty. The chairman relied upon them heavily, but not because he looked to them for guidance on what to push and how much to push for. Rather, he decided pretty much on his own, though with verification from various sources, which research area could use attention and money. With his extraordinary political sensitivity as regards the mood of the House, and against the backdrop of the broader political situation, he would decide what increase he thought he could get his colleagues to go along with for medical research. Then he would invite witnesses and extract from them testimony most strongly supportive of his strategy. By the time his bill came to the House floor, Colonel Quinn had let a few of the chairman's colleagues not on the subcommittee know what increase for NIH he was asking for, and they would be standing by to say a word of support.[42] Each year Fogarty's own Irish Brigade—Eddie Boland of Massachusetts, John Rooney of New York, Mike Kirwan of Ohio, Leon Gavin of Pennsylvania, John Monaghan of Connecticut, Leonore Sullivan of Missouri, Florence Dwyer of New Jersey, and Jim O'Hara of Michigan—rose to commend the able, expert, hard-working Gentleman from Rhode Island for his vision and his leadership, and to support strongly the increases he proposed and which the most outstanding medicine men in the country endorsed.[43]

The communications system he helped provide was what, to Colonel Quinn, made the greatest difference. The testimony of "medical romantics" like Farber and DeBakey was important, as grist for the mill, but it took political energy to get it grinding.[44] Complimenting chairman Fogarty on his having led the Congress to supply funds for a mental health personnel training program some years before, during his testimony in 1959, Mike Gorman heard the compliment returned. "It was your idea," said Fogarty. Gorman would concede that, but he reminded the chairman: "I had no vote when the markup session came." [45]

In private, however, the professional lobbyists and their backers, like the medical professionals, take pride in their catalytic role. Mary Lasker acknowledges that she was John Fogarty's first tutor in medical research. Florence Mahoney influenced Senator Hill to take the Senate subcommittee chairmanship.

In the end, they all needed each other, even as principals in a play need other principals as well as a supporting cast. Clearly, though policy prerogatives had been claimed by Congress and political power seemed to be centered there, it was shared power, and power requiring the bolstering authority of professional expertise. Nor would it do any good simply for those who proximately made policy—the chairmen of the Labor-HEW appropriations subcommittees, their ranking opposites, and a few executive branch officials—to do so unless those who must carry it out, the scientists and physicians, were willing partners. Meanwhile, outsiders pushing the Cause—medical men, professional lobbyists, and their singleminded backers—followed the classic description, in substance and style, of the role they were all engaged in: "Interest group leaders influence the proximate policy maker through persuasion. They try to persuade him that what they want is what he too thinks is best—or that what he should realize is best is what they want." [46]

That the roles were sometimes reversed, with the "proximate policy maker" persuading the interest group leaders—or the working scientists—that what he wanted was best for them too, is not so surprising, at least to those who have watched legislators' relationships with lobbyists at close range. What is remarkable is that two other professional types, the university administrator and the practicing physician, seemed to be ignored in the course of policy development. Only occasionally a department chairman or medical school dean would ask, or be asked, to appear before the committees and offer counsel as to the best way in which and the best pace at which to proceed with the medical research enterprise.[47]

The American Medical Association, meanwhile, seemed to have no contribution to make. For a long time it was as though the organization which represented most of the thousands of practicing physicians had vacated the field of medical research policy. Having so long fought the federal government's potential involvement in most other health spheres—medical care, health insurance, the training of physicians through scholarships and direct support of teaching in medical schools—it might be natural that, as a political strategy, it would not also fight federal efforts in medical research, which in any case could be considered a much less potent threat. Ultimately the Association came to realize that there was a major and ironic incongruity in the fact that the organization claiming as a cardinal tenet the advancement of good health for all citizens had had nothing to do with the greatest effort of the century to make possible the attainment of that goal. Finally, in June 1964, the organization's board of trustees impaneled a Commission on Research.[48]

In a statement released at the White House Conference on Health on November 3–4, 1965, Dr. James Z. Appel stated: "No one is more aware than the physician of the overwhelming importance of scientific research as an aspect of our national life. Without it, none of medicine's triumphs would be ours today. No one is more concerned that research be continued in the future on a wise and prudent course guaranteeing continued progress in the medical field." The AMA Commission on Research would gauge "the scope of the current effort, particularly in relation to medicine and medical education." It would seek "to determine the impact of present programs." [49]

In February 1967, the AMA Commission's report emerged. Admitting that the AMA had never "unequivocally endorsed Federal research grants as a whole," but claiming to have "endorsed and supported specific medical research legislation" and to have "never opposed any Federal appropriation for the support of medical research," the Commission concurred "in the general belief that the current level of adequacy and excellence of our biomedical research resources has never before been equalled." (It did speculate that some mediocre research had probably been supported, though.) It recommended to the board of trustees that "the American Medical Association should support in general the Federal biomedical research program" and that "the programs of the National Institutes of Health should be recognized for their contributions to the National biomedical research effort." [50]

Perhaps Congress, and its counselors—scientists and administrators of the National Institutes of Health, other professional medical advisers, professional lobbyists, and lay supporters— were glad to have the American Medical Association's support, however late, however qualified, and however grudging. Meanwhile, they had together built a great national medical research enterprise of which the central component alone, NIH, was spending over $1 billion annually.

Still, new friends were important, especially if there had been some dropouts from the Crusade. In their zeal, the professionals had come close to alienating some of the drug manufacturers, by pushing for increased spending by NIH on the development of drugs that might effectively combat cancer and mental illness. The problem was that some pharmaceutical houses were already investing their own money in the field, and they resented what they thought was an attempt to take from them profitable patentable drug possibilities and, under the rules of government sponsorship, put research results at the disposal even of their competitors who had invested none of their own resources.

Mike Gorman stated the position of the citizens groups:

> Several drug companies have complained to me that the evaluation of cancer compounds by the National Cancer Service Center is an infringement on the sacred right of private enterprise.
>
> Why, they argue, should a group of federally appointed scientists decide what anti-cancer compound is effective against a certain type of cancer? My answer, sir, is a very simple one—because human life is at stake.
>
> Some of us who are testifying today have carried the battle for use of tranquilizing drugs for 5 years in the face of

very bitter resistance. We have done so not because we are interested in the profits or patents of the drug houses, but because we are interested in human life.[51]

Karl Bamback, whom Gorman had identified as the "Washington lobbyist of the American Drug Manufacturers Association," answered with an argument and a label of his own: "The reason many research authorities, including some at NIH, as well as in the pharmaceutical industry, do not favor an industry-government contract program to produce even more tranquilizing drugs is that they fear the net result would harm the total research effort of the country. The pharmaceutical industry would prefer to carry out such research with its own money."

Nor should the Congress be fooled about who was getting paid to do what. Bamback reminded Senator Hill that "some of the spokesmen for the so-called citizens groups, which I recently referred to, are really professional lobbyists." [52]

VIII   The Dangers of Political Success

President Eisenhower viewed the government's expanding involvement in medical research ambivalently. Although he acceded on more than one occasion to those favoring ever greater increases, he could not get over the fear that the enterprise was being pushed too fast.

On the other hand, Ike apparently felt at the beginning of his presidency that fiscal stringencies were to be applied somewhat less rigorously to programs directly affecting the health and welfare of human beings than to other categories, an approach that surprised and chagrined some of his fiscally conservative associates. Joseph Dodge, Eisenhower's first Budget Director, thought that President Truman had loaded the budget he left his successor with every dollar and programmatic frill he could. Dodge saw his role, he told his young assistant, William Carey, as that of "dismantling the Christmas tree." He was stunned when the President replaced his revised figures for certain domestic health and education programs with the higher ones in the Truman budget. The President explained to his budget director that he wanted the agency responsible for "people programs" to be a showpiece.[1]

HEW Secretary Marion Folsom had perceived this interest of the President and was naturally inclined to push it. When called over to the Budget Bureau in September 1955 to discuss his proposed departmental budget for fiscal 1956, Folsom was cordially welcomed. Any friend and associate of Secretary of the Treasury George Humphrey was obviously a friend of the Bureau. The Bureau assumed, suggested Director Percival Brundage, that the Secretary would be amenable to any cuts in his budget which the Bureau thought necessary. Folsom upset that assumption by remarking that, having left the Treasury

Department, his was a different role now; and he retrieved a quotation from the President to the effect that programs for the improvement of the well-being of citizens were to be given special treatment. His own assumption being that the President meant what he said on that point, Folsom was not going to automatically accept any proposed cuts in his budget by the Bureau. In fact, he intended to recommend, and if necessary fight for, increases over the preliminary budget estimates.[2]

Eisenhower backed Folsom's proposed increases for NIH in 1956 and 1957, and in 1960 he decided not to veto the HEW budget with its heavy increases in money for NIH insisted upon by Congress. Still, he remarked to Dr. Farber, a lot of his doctor friends had told him that the government was pushing medical research too fast.

Informal evaluations had not supported that belief. Nor had the formal report commissioned by Secretary Folsom in 1957 and delivered in 1958 by a task force of consultants headed by the former Surgeon General of the Army, General Stanhope Bayne-Jones. Though subsequent departmental budget requests did not reflect it, the Bayne-Jones report put the medical research effort on a plane of high importance and gave the National Institutes of Health good marks for its central role in the enterprise.[3]

Some in Congress shared the President's ambivalence. The paean of praise that greeted the annual presentation of the proposed NIH appropriations suggests a genuine interest, even a pride, on the part of colleagues of Hill, Thye, Fogarty, and Laird in what was acknowledged to be a successful example of congressional policy initiative. But the growth was so rapid that it made even some friends a little nervous. Polls might show that the American people favored medical research and generally thought that more should be spent, but their elected representatives in Congress are, despite occasional evidence to the contrary, very anxious to be sure that monies from the public purse are well spent and efficiently used, that there is no waste, no gross mistakes. Aside from defeat at the polls, Congressmen are scared of nothing so much as a bust after a boom, and they like good management as much as they dislike controversy.

Senator Leverett Saltonstall, the ranking Republican member of the Senate Appropriations Committee, felt need of reassurance, in 1958, that the committee—which always went along with the subcommittee's recommendations—was making the right decision in increasing medical research funds at so rapid a pace. He thought the Committee needed outside, objective counsel about whether the funds provided were being efficiently used, and he suggested to the subcommittee in his ex officio role that such an evaluation be made before the 1960 appropriations were taken up.

Senator Hill, gracious as always, was glad to oblige the senior Senator from Massachusetts. He thought the question should be put more generally—whether funds for medical research and NIH were at the proper level—but it was nonetheless a good idea.[4] He asked Boisfeullet Jones, who was Vice President for Medical Affairs of Emory University, to head a committee of consultants "to determine whether the funds provided by the Government for research in dread diseases are sufficient and efficiently spent in the best interests of the research for which they were designated."[5]

Hill had not previously known Jones well,[6] although he knew his reputation as an able university administrator and a knowledgeable person on the subject of medical schools, their activities, and their finances. Others named to the Jones Committee were old friends in the cause of medical research: Dr. DeBakey, Sidney Farber, Harry Lyons of the Dental Association, General Sarnoff, Cornelius Traeger of the Multiple Sclerosis Society, and Cecil Wittson. Hill told Jones he wanted a searching inquiry, and suggested no obvious or particular outcomes. But friends of the Cause had a quorum.

The opportunity which membership on the Committee of

Consultants provided for those regular outside advisers to the Congress who had consistently urged rapid, solid expansion of the government's biomedical research effort was a rare one. Ordinarily, particular interest groups must take their chances with the rest of them, figuring out a way to gain access to the policy maker, competing for time to make their case, and often having to struggle against opposing interest groups. The medical research lobby not only had no opposite number, but the opportunity to present its case had already been elevated, guaranteed, institutionalized by the congressional committees that needed persuasion. They were high-class burglars, admitted Mike Gorman, who walked right in the front door and were cordially welcomed by those holding the resources they were after.[7] Now if the Jones Committee reached agreement on major points, that would be tantamount to passing approval on one's own grant.

Always the medical professionals and the professional lobbyists had to document their pleas with figures, case studies, medical judgments, and predictions. Their success was not based simply on emotion and desire and empathy; rather they had to sell and convince on the basis of analysis, even if the potential buyer was generally disposed to spend. If, as Charles Lindblom suggests, "partisan analysis" is the main source of power of interest groups,[8] this new opportunity was one to solidify what was already considerable, possibly unique, power. What was involved here was an invitation to highly skilled practitioners of partisan analysis to perform that analysis for a group of clients, most of whom hoped the analysis would be partisan, and the rest of whom would be satisfied just because it was analysis.

The Jones Committee made its report to the Senate Appropriations Subcommittee in May 1960. In the course of its analysis it had relied upon "100 expert witnesses" as well as numerous documents and reports, and it had new information that had been developed at its request. "It reached its judgments after extended discussion by unanimous agreement." Its main conclusions were: "as a whole, the funds appropriated by Congress for the support of research on major disease problems have been expended by Federal agencies with remarkable efficiency; . . . the National Institutes of Health, which Congress has made the principal instrument for disbursement of funds for medical research," have been extremely successful in maintaining "consistent high standards for the research supported," gaining "the confidence of the scientific community," and upholding "the traditional freedom of both institutions and investigators." Further, despite the generosity of the Congress in providing increased funds to support research over the last 15 years, "they have not kept pace with new opportunities in research which have developed, largely as the result of the very advances which the funds expended in the past have generated." In general, the Committee felt that "the great advances already forthcoming from this program justify the expectation that, through medical research, the span of useful, enjoyable life can be still further lengthened, and that the benefit to society of longer, healthier and more productive lives will be far greater than the cost of the research required to reach that goal." [9]

The Committee was even more specific about what the needs were. They recommended increases in the President's budget for NIH for fiscal 1961 in the amount of $264 million and specified what areas should receive the increases.[10]

The Senate committee "accepted the recommendations of the consultants as being sound." They approved appropriations for NIH in precisely the amount recommended. Further, warned the subcommittee's report to the Senate, "those increases should be regarded not as a maximum level but as the floor from which further advances will be made in years to come." [11] The final figure agreed upon by Congress that year—the last Eisenhower budget—was $547 million.

Many persons thought that with the coming of the Democratic administration of John F. Kennedy two things would happen: first they expected that the new administration, in contrast to its predecessor, would be truly generous toward medical research. And by contrast it was. The first Kennedy budget included an increase for NIH of $40 million, the largest dollar increase ever proposed for medical research by a President and the largest percentage increase proposed since 1955 when Marion Folsom persuaded President Eisenhower that the need and the competence were there.

The second thing some expected to happen was that the Democratic Congress, out of appreciation of the President's leadership in the premises, would defer to his proposed budget. There was a lingering suspicion that the nonpartisan congressional committee approach to medical research, which had principally involved Democrats raising a Republican President's budgets, and Republicans at least once raising a Democratic President's budget, would crumble when a liberal Democratic President dealt with a liberal Democratic Congress. Fogarty and Hill laid that suspicion to rest in the spring and summer of 1961 when they got the Congress to approve appropriations for NIH in the amount of $783 million, $155 million more than the President had asked for. Representative Melvin Laird, urging the House to go along with the subcommittee rather than with the new President, reminded his colleagues on both sides of the aisle that in its nonpartisan approach to medical research the committee had frequently gone beyond the executive budget, indeed had usually done so when the budget figure, in the committee's judgment, was inadequate. Unfortunately, said Laird, this was not one of those years when the President's request is sufficient.[12] Furthermore, the committee blamed the low budget request for NIH on one of its favorite targets, the Budget Bureau: NIH had asked for $641 million and that figure had been accepted by the Department of Health, Education and Welfare. "The Committee has tried to determine from the Secretary, from the Surgeon General, and from the Director of the National Institutes of Health, why the Bureau of the Budget reduced this request by $58 million. Since no other specific reasons have been given the Committee, it can only conclude that this was purely an arbitrary reduction." [13] Its recommendations to the House having always been based on deep, probing, professional judgments and nonpartisan reasoning, naturally the committee would not accept the Bureau's arbitrary action. It accepted instead the $641 million figure that NIH and HEW had suggested in the first place.

The Senate, still riding the crest of the wave made by its Committee of Consultants, added another $200 million; the final figure was the usual compromise approximately halfway between the amount proposed by the House and the amount proposed by the Senate. The figure the Conference Committee of the House and Senate agreed upon was $738 million. It caused problems when it was presented to the House again, but that record-breaking sum was finally accepted.[14]

Senator William Proxmire (D., Wis.), programmatic liberal and staunch fiscal conservative, was incredulous. He could understand why, he intimated, when the executive presented static or otherwise unsatisfactory budgets for medical research, the Congress might wish to increase those funds. But now, Proxmire argued, a different situation prevailed. President Kennedy was a sensitive and compassionate man, and he had already added more than $37 million to the NIH budget. He thought the Senate should defer to the new President.[15]

The subcommittee chairman saw it differently: "I have the same respect for the President of the United States as does the Senator from Wisconsin. The President of the United States has not had the time or the opportunity to hear the testimony, to get the facts, to know the complexities as have the members of the Committee on Appropriations of the House and the Committee on Appropriations of the Senate." [16]

President Kennedy well understood the potency of medical research as a Cause, and he recognized the Congress' pride of authorship. He had himself been a special pleader at least once.

In 1955 the junior Senator from Massachusetts had lauded the subcommittee for "in almost every case increasing substantially the amount of money available for the National Institutes of Health." It was, he had said on the Senate floor, "most appropriate for the subcommittee to do so." He was concerned about one item for which there was no proposed increase by the subcommittee:

> Senator Kennedy: It is my understanding that no additional money was appropriated for the National Institutes of Health division of research grants . . .
> Senator Hill: What amount would the Senator suggest?
> Kennedy: The backlog of projects which are approved calls for $1 million. I think that if one-half of that amount could be provided, it would make a tremendous difference . . .
> Hill: I have not consulted with the Senator on this matter, and I cannot speak for the Committee. However, so far as I am concerned, as chairman of the subcommitee, I shall be happy to suggest that the Senate agree to an amendment and shall certainly take it to conference, if the Senator should see fit to offer it.
> Kennedy: I shall do so.[17]

The Kennedy amendment, adding another half-million dollars, passed on a voice vote.

But Jack Kennedy knew the men involved as well as the atmosphere. The President thought he could persuade his former House colleague, his fellow Democratic Irishman from New England, to be more reasonable. One story goes that the President called John Fogarty down to the White House shortly after he had sent up to the Hill the HEW budget and before Fogarty had set in motion that process which, unless checked, would probably produce increases for NIH. Fogarty somehow knew what the President wanted to ask him, and he wanted to be prepared. Kennedy suggested to Fogarty that, in view of new executive thrust, there was no need for the House to raise the figures and asked Fogarty's cooperation. The chairman replied that he wanted to cooperate with his leader and would try to do so; the only problem was, just that morning he had advised the House in spontaneous remarks that in reviewing the proposed NIH budget it seemed to him to be once again deficient, and he had put his colleagues on notice that the subcommittee might raise those figures.

Nonetheless, a year later, in 1963, the House and the Congress as a whole reduced a President's budget for medical research for the first time in decades, cutting the executive budget estimates from $930 million to $912 million. Had the President, after all, persuaded his zealous friend John Fogarty to defer to the Administration in the matter of NIH budgets?

Various reasons were offered for the new congressional posture that year. John Fogarty told the House that the reason was simply that, for the first time in years, the administration proposals were "soundly conceived." [18] They certainly were progressive in monetary terms; the proposed budget called for an appropriation for NIH of $930 million, $150 million more than what had been requested the previous year and more than $130 million than Congress had appropriated. There were, however, a couple of other factors. Congressman Laird explained one of them, reminding his colleagues of the situation the previous year when "the other body" had added tremendous additional sums on top of the additions already approved by the House. He had favored the House increase but thought the Senate had gone too far. "I brought back the conference report on this bill in disagreement, and made a motion to recommit the conference report . . . We lost that roll call by some 17 votes . . . I hope that this year, if the other body will not yield to our position, that we will be able to get back those 17 votes we lost last year and keep this program at an adequate but proper level as is proposed in the bill now before the House." [19]

Not only John Fogarty but Lister Hill got the message. There were repercussions in the appropriations subcommittee of the Senate as well as that of the House. Senator Proxmire had introduced an amendment to restore the figure suggested by the President and had drawn an impressive array of support. There were liberal Democrats (Paul Douglas and Joseph Clark), conservative Democrats (James Eastland and Frank Laushe), liberal Republicans (John Sherman Cooper and Frank Case) and conservative Republicans (Henry Dvorak and Karl Mundt). The vote crossed party, sectional, and philosophical lines, with some of each category on each side of the issue. Happily for Senator Hill, 46 of his colleagues voted with him, while only 32 supported the Proxmire move.[20] One thing that particularly disturbed Hill was that the ranking member of the appropriations committee, Leverett Saltonstall, voted against him. And when members of one's committee break the bond of nonpartisan unanimity, trouble lies ahead.

Norris Cotton, Hill's ranking opposite on the subcommittee, thus found Hill amenable to going slower the following year. He extracted a promise from Hill not to push for sizable increases; in return, Cotton would keep the tradition of nonpartisan unity.[21] In 1963, the Senate Committee approved the budget exactly as submitted by the President; what had become the annual Proxmire effort to reduce the NIH appropriations failed by a vote of 58 to 27. (Hill got more of his colleagues to the floor for the vote; Proxmire's support began slipping away.) For the first time, the final congressional appropriation for NIH was less than what the executive had asked for.

Whether they came from within or without, the occasional attacks on Congress' effort to build a great medical research enterprise had been based on simple concepts of fiscal conservatism. The Budget Bureau added an "executive planning" argument to the fiscal one; but from the time the AMA dropped its professed fear of federal control, most of those who opposed congressional increases did so because they just couldn't believe that *that* much money was necessary, because they thought such rapid growth inevitably meant inefficiency and probably waste.

One of the formulas advanced by Senator William Proxmire to reduce appropriations for the several institutes of NIH was to cut the figures back to the lowest estimate of need, whether it had been suggested by NIH, HEW, Budget Bureau, House Appropriations Subcommittee, citizen witnesses, or Senate Appropriations Subcommittee.[22] (He apparently thought such a formula might have more appeal than simply accepting the Budget Bureau's estimates, though they were always the lowest figures.) Senators Prescott Bush (R., Conn.) and Styles Bridges occasionally wanted to reduce the aggregate appropriation for all agencies in the Labor-HEW group by a given percentage or a given dollar amount, to be equally spread across those agencies.[23] Congressman Frank Bow of Ohio sometimes made similar proposals to achieve lower budgets,[24] and Senator Everett Dirksen often moved to recommit the Labor-HEW appropriations bill with instructions to the committee to come back with lower figures generally.[25] Senator Gordon Allott (R., Colo.) supported the Dirksen motion in 1960; as a member of the subcommittee, his complaint was a single, general one: "We must face the fact that we are spending too much money." [26]

There is little wonder that such an approach so often failed, especially when it is contrasted with the approach of those proposing greater funds for medical research. The proponents documented their case disease category by disease category, institute by institute, program by program, on the basis of specific (if onesided) testimony and documentation. The opponents down through the years simply proposed reductions or rollbacks in various percentages and on the basis of general formulas that may have been fiscally sensible but were judgmentally arbitrary. True, the political atmosphere was conducive to medical research expansion and discouraging to those who wanted to go slower. But it was not quite so irrational a state as Senator

Proxmire painted, in which, he complained, if you don't vote for increases you are thought of as "the fast friend of cancer, the buddy of heart disease." [27] His was a more difficult role than Lister Hill's, but in the end he simply didn't make a strong enough case on sufficiently specific grounds.

One would think that, if the figures presented by citizens witnesses were inflated, they could have been punctured by professional judgments on the other side. If the evidence of significant medical breakthroughs were sparse and the descriptions of general progress vague, one would think that, with some homework and some outside help, the picture could be put in less dramatic and possibly less compelling perspective. Never did any of those who opposed the policy of increasing support for biomedical science—expanding the number of medical scientists supported and trained with federal funds with a view toward reducing the effects of "dread human disease"—argue that medical progress was not being made, or even that medical progress was not being made at a rate commensurate with the rate of increase in support funds. They could not reasonably argue the former, and perhaps they could not argue the latter, on the basis of hard evidence. But they could have, with a less simplistic, more than hortatory approach, made a more effective stand.

It was Lawrence H. Fountain (D., N.C.), chairman of the Intergovernmental Relations Subcommittee of the House Government Operations Committee, who finally found a chink in the armor. The soft underbelly of the medical research empire, he discovered, was in the area of administration and management.

By 1960, the National Institutes of Health were spending more than half of their half-billion-dollar budget to support research performed in universities and nonprofit institutions throughout the country through grants. Over 11,500 projects were under way that year on a broad spectrum of biomedical research endeavors. They were undertaken in more than 400 institutions of higher learning, as well as a much smaller number of nonprofit, nonuniversity organizations. Approximately 200 of all universities and medical schools whose faculty and staff members were involved in federally supported research received 90 percent of all federal research funds. As a rough summary, in 1960 approximately 200 universities and medical schools were awarded $250 million for the support of more than 10,000 research projects from the National Institutes of Health.[28]

That this enormous endeavor was producing specific medical progress was accepted by most. That it represented the greatest medical research enterprise in the history of the world was occasionally mentioned by some. And many persons in the university world and some persons in the federal government believed that it constituted a massive program of federal aid to education. It was not an untroubled activity, and tensions between individual institutional performers of medical research and the sponsoring federal agencies occasionally arose. But generally both sponsors and performers thought that they, and society at large, were gaining much out of the enterprise, and no one directly involved would have thought of scaling it down on philosophical or fiscal grounds.

With an operation that big and that far-flung, neither was anyone greatly surprised that problems of administration and management existed and could easily be identified. Least surprised of all was Dr. James Shannon, director of NIH and Chancellor of the Empire's Exchequer. The manner in which and reasons for which the enterprise had grown so big so fast had not encouraged, indeed had made very difficult, simultaneous expansion of sophisticated management capability within NIH. Congress wanted money spent on research by scientists, not supervision of research by administrative types. Similarly, while Congress voted regularly for increasing dollars to be spent in this area, they also voted regularly to hold down the number of federal employees generally, a matter which directly affected this area. As far as potential research administrators could tell, it was personally more advantageous financially to remain in research-performing institutions than to join the sponsoring government agency to help manage the enterprise from the center.

Other potential management difficulties stemmed from continuing apprehensions of government interference on the part of nongovernment researchers, and continuing sensitivities of government administrators to that concern. Furthermore, with the executive branch of the government not offering leadership in setting a reasonable and consistent pace for expanding the research effort, and with that leadership consequently devolving on Congress, the result was that "for the operating agency . . . planning is always after the fact of the budget accomplishment rather than before it." [29]

Congressman Fountain delicately approached the job of probing potential weak spots. His committee would not, he said, "consciously do anything which will impair the effectiveness of [NIH] programs." It was simply that he wanted to help the agency remedy management deficiencies. Thus the Fountain Committee proceeded with its charge, "the responsibility of studying the operation of NIH with a view to determining its economy and efficiency." And though he intended to be gentle, he offered the following caution to the NIH management and their friends inside and outside Congress: "While I fully appreciate that the support of scientific research—particularly in academic institutions—is a very sensitive and complex operation, this does not relieve NIH of its responsibility of its accountability for the prudent expenditure of public funds." [30]

It was the discrete area of research grants management that the Fountain Committee began to probe in 1959. But it was the larger task of reining in the total enterprise that the Committee seemed to have in mind. The Kennedy Administration was being terribly liberal in its budgetary attitude toward NIH, remarked Fountain; and the add-ons urged by the House and Senate Appropriations Subcommittees thus seemed especially unnecessary. Members of Congress, he suggested, were becoming increasingly concerned; a number of members had asked him, with regard to the 1962 appropriations bill for the Departments of Labor and Health, Education and Welfare whether they ought to vote for that measure with its proposed $60 million extra for NIH. Members usually accepted "on faith" the recommendations of the appropriations subcommittee, not only because they wanted to favor medical research progress, but because that bill, like most others, had annually come to include something for everyone—there was "something in everybody's district." Fountain quoted approvingly an editorial in the *Washington Star* complaining that NIH was being force-fed by Congress, and especially by Fogarty.[31]

The first major Fountain Committee report, issued in April 1961, was mild. "The Committee found that NIH is not adequately organized to administer the grant programs with maximum effectiveness." It offered 13 recommendations which it felt would substantially improve the grants operations of the Institutes.[32]

NIH had cooperated with the Fountain Committee in providing its staff with all information requested during the examination of management practices. Now it reacted officially to the criticisms with grace. Most of the recommendations were "entirely acceptable"; Dr. Shannon complimented chairman Fountain on "a searching and constructive inquiry into the growing and complex set of activities administered by the National Institutes of Health." Surgeon General Luther Terry told Fountain that he thought the "study and report rendered a service to the national research effort." [33]

Somewhat nervously, the appropriations subcommittee leaders watched. They played down the suggested weaknesses, as well as ignoring the significance of the larger thrust. Representative Laird commented in 1961, in urging House approval of the subcommittee bill with all its increases: "I went over the [Fountain Committee] report and I did not find the report very critical." [34]

But critical or not, it was the entering wedge into the complicated, Congress-dominated policy system which had succeeded for almost a decade in directing the development of "the most effective research program in the world." Based on explicit criticisms stemming from focused examination of specific aspects of the medical research enterprise, Congressman Fountain accomplished what no other critic, in Congress or the executive branch, had been able to accomplish. His was not a lethal blow to the Cause, by any means, but for a time it was staggering.

Fountain's job had been made easier because the leaders of the march had, in their zeal, overextended themselves: in carrying NIH from a budget of $400 million in 1961 to $738 million in 1962, ignoring President Kennedy's suggested level of $583 million, the subcommittee chairmen (especially Senator Hill, who didn't seem to want to let Fogarty get ahead of him as a budget raiser) had given a set of nerves to some of their friends as well as evidence of irresponsibility to their potential opponents. In his opinion, said Fountain, "had an all out effort been made to reduce these funds, notwithstanding the very wonderful job which Congressman Fogarty did, there would have been . . . a reduction of those funds." [35]

If superextravagance in 1961 on the part of congressional friends of medical research was a special invitation for the sort of criticism the Fountain Committee produced, the reaction of NIH and some of its newly vocal friends in 1962 and thereafter exacerbated and prolonged the effects. In reviewing its first report in a special series of hearings with the Fountain Committee in March 1962, Dr. Shannon, credited by many with being a good politician as well as a superb science administrator, committed what is perhaps the cardinal sin of legislative-executive etiquette. Apparently annoyed that the Fountain Committee intended to persist, in its oversight activities, in its insistence that Shannon and his NIH administrative colleagues carry out their recommendations (after all, had not he told the committee that he would carry out those that were proper and practicable?) Shannon suggested to the committee that it was pursuing a minor theme, or worse. The only truly important thing said Shannon, falling back on that cliché-conviction dear to the hearts of established, well-funded scientists, was in selecting the right man. "This is the point at which really significant administrative actions designed to make programs efficient and productive are taken. Selection of good men and good ideas —and the rejection of the inferior—is the key. All subsequent administrative actions having to do with the adjustment of budgets, and so forth, are essentially trivial in relation to this basic selection process." [36]

Senator Hill (and Congressmen Fogarty and Laird) might have agreed privately with Dr. Shannon that the Fountain Committee was poking into less than crucial matters and was muddying the whole stream in the process. But Hill was reportedly furious with Shannon for his injudicious use of language. Hill knew that the way to win and keep friends, and sidetrack possible detractors, was by being ever gracious and cooperative. You avoided confrontations, even avoided controversies if you could (and Hill's colleagues say that when possible he avoided taking formal votes in committee);[37] under no circumstances did you question the motives or the seriousness of anyone's objections to the way you wanted to proceed.[38] And if those rules govern relations among members of Congress, they should operate even more strongly between executive branch officials and congressional committee chairmen.

The congressional roles of oversight, auditing, and investigating—which some political scientists say Congress ought to be limited to and others say Congress already largely limits itself to—are not unimportant. Moreover, it is perhaps natural that Congress performs such functions more readily than it engages in broad policy development because review, investigation, and analysis of existing policies and programs is by far the easier task. Further, modification of policy may result from conscientious execution of oversight, so that the role is not necessarily unconstructive. Often, however, it is unimaginative, as is any pursuit where the focus is on operational detail rather than grand design and purpose.

Shannon's vision of the grand design is one of the factors that enabled him to serve so effectively as director general of the medical research enterprise, sitting between those on one side who fashioned a policy they believed and expected would bring the American people into a new age of good health and long life, of freedom from fear of disease; and on the other, those scientists who pursued truth, who pushed back the frontiers of knowledge bit by bit, who day to day engaged in the meticulous and fascinating effort to find new answers to old or new, particular or general, scientific problems. The two groups did not unreservedly trust each other, although their mutual dependency was crucial. The policy makers and many of their advisers thought the scientists could pursue the goal with greater alacrity and sharper focus; the researchers thought the policy initiators did not fully understand the scientific process. Dr. Alvin Weinberg, director of the Oak Ridge National Laboratory, has commented that he doubts there are many researchers who work on basic research because they prefer that to a specific attempt to find a cure for cancer; it's just that they don't know enough to direct their whole energies to that single purpose.[39]

Dr. Shannon's concept was that once the great medical research enterprise was constructed—grounded in solid, basic knowledge, embracing first-rate scientists following many approaches—it was possible that now-secret answers to actual, specific biophysical problems affecting man would be uncovered. Only a person with the capacity for such a broad view, and normally with the capacity for verbally reconciling the differing emphases, could be successful in carrying out what had come to be national policy. A smaller mind or more obvious partisan of one or the other potentially conflicting views would have inevitably offended if not alienated essential members of the enterprise.

Furthermore, Shannon was proud of his administrative approach to the burgeoning national system. The more Congress appropriated for medical research, the stricter the criteria he imposed to insure against waste. Congress understood this, he said, and the approach was one of the key reasons the House and Senate committees felt comfortable in continuing their largesse. Every year NIH turned some of the money appropriated to it back to the Treasury because the bioscience managers felt it could not be used efficiently or with certainty about results.

Thus the proud administrator of a magnificent enterprise, the man of broad vision who felt that his own capacity for self-criticism made unnecessary criticism by others, although he tried to be understanding of the congressional novices who were entering this difficult, complex field, ultimately became impatient with them and suggested they turn their spotlight away from incidental activities, from trivial considerations, because it was distracting attention from center stage.

That the Fountain Committee was offended, and probably angry, is suggested by the attention its subsequent report gave Dr. Shannon's pointed remark. In its June 1962 report it responded equally pointedly:

> The committee agrees that the selection of good investigators and good projects is vital to productive scientific research, but the effective management of grants is also a fundamental responsibility of a Government agency charged with administering grant programs.
>
> The committee takes strong exception to the view expressed by NIH that all administrative actions subsequent to the selection of grant projects are "essentially trivial" in relation to the basic selection process. The selection

process and grant management are essential and complementary parts of NIH research support. Excellence is required of both.[40]

Further, Shannon's summary of his approach to his job gave the Committee an opening to bring the broader charge its chairman had earlier hinted he wanted to make:

It appears that Congress has been overzealous in appropriating money for health research. The conclusion is inescapable, from a study of NIH's loose administrative practices, that the pressure for spending increasingly large appropriations has kept NIH from giving adequate attention to basic management problems. The committee expects NIH to give high priority at this time to the task of correcting its management deficiencies and strengthening its capability for the effective and efficient operation of these vital health programs.[41]

The next time Congress considered appropriations for the National Institutes of Health, in 1963 (fiscal 1964), the budget proposed by the executive was scaled down by $15 million.

Simultaneously, the President of the United States asked for a wholesale review of the national medical research effort as embodied in the activities of the National Institutes of Health, activities which represented "direct financial support of forty percent of the nation's health research; a pattern of legal arrangemen's with more than one thousand universities and medical schools, involving more than 17,000 separate grants; growth by a factor of ten in eight years; an annual budget approaching the billion dollar level." [42]

Joseph D. Cooper, who has followed NIH growth and frequently commented upon the environment that produced it, attributes the creation of the Woolridge Committee in significant part to Congressman Fountain's activities. For although "the Fountain Committee had not gone very deeply into appraisals of scientific quality, it had raised questions which some felt had to be resolved one way or the other."[43]

The assassination of President Kennedy interrupted the new evaluation. But early in 1964, with the specific endorsement of President Lyndon Johnson, a 13-man committee headed by Dr. Dean E. Woolridge began "to study how NIH spends its approximately billion dollar budget, to judge whether the American people are getting their money's worth from the expenditure, and to recommend any changes in organization or procedure that would in our opinion increase the effectiveness of the program."[44] This time there were no members of the Committee who could be said to be faithful champions of the Cause. Aside from Dr. Woolridge, there were seven university officials plus one university board chairman, a foundation president, two business executives, and the Commissioner of Health of New York City.

The Woolridge Committee spent one year making a "firsthand investigation of NIH activities," using 77 scientists and administrators who "participated extensively in the data-gathering and evaluation." More than 600 NIH-funded scientists were visited, as were 150 institutional administrators.[45]

In February 1965, the Committee presented its findings to the President. "The first and probably the most important general conclusion [was] that the activities of the National Institutes of Health are essentially sound and that its budget of approximately one billion dollars a year is, on the whole, being spent wisely and well in the public interest." What was in need of strengthening, said the Committee, were "the organization and procedures of NIH."[46]

The policy goals described by Woolridge were somewhat at variance with the statutory purposes stated by those legislative acts creating the various institutes and giving NIH its research authority and charge. Categorical disease labels, said the Committee, "in the titles of the major organizational units of NIH suggests more of an orientation than actually exists." It gave the NIH management great credit for "making a scientifically inappropriate organizational structure an effective arrangement for performing its real mission." But in pursuing its "primary *de facto* mission . . . of the stimulation and support of a very broad range of health-related or biomedical research," the National Institutes of Health got high marks.[47]

Put another way, national medical research policy, in the Woolridge Committee's view, was to concentrate on a wide range of rather freely performed basic research and employ directed developmental research aimed at conquering cancer and other specific diseases only when there was relative certainty of promising results. So defined, the policy was sensible and well aimed; the NIH program which operated under it was sound. The Woolridge Committee recommended continued support for both.

While others sniped at the Woolridge Committee's operating procedures and questioned the documentation of some of its conclusions and recommendations (and while the Fountain Committee probably felt its position on management weaknesses had been bolstered), the congressional sponsors of continued expansion of the national medical research activity, with the National Institutes of Health at its center, found the report most reassuring, even vindicating. After two years of reducing the BOB estimates for NIH in the wake of the Fountain Committee reports, the House Appropriations Subcommittee once more moved the figures upward, adding $12 million to the $867 million proposed by the Administration.[48]

Senator Hill praised the Woolridge Committee and its findings in presenting to the Senate in August 1965 his subcommittee's proposed appropriations for NIH for the fiscal year that had already begun. He quoted excerpts from the report of the "distinguished board." [49] Most important for his purposes was the following paragraph.

In brief, we consider the NIH program to be sound and recommend its continued support. Its $1 billion budget is not high, when compared to the more than thirty billion dollars a year the American public pays for assorted health services; the money is on the whole competently and efficiently employed on a broad spectrum of health related research; lessons from the past history of science, supported by the current acceleration of medical discovery, strongly suggest a satisfactory future payoff. Furthermore, as discoveries are made in the life sciences, new opportunities will be created for health research, and these too should be exploited with the enthusiasm and vigor which has distinguished the NIH program during the past decade. We feel that the Congress in particular deserves considerable credit for its past support of this kind of farsighted program. We suspect that there are few, if any, one billion dollar segments of the Federal budget that are buying more valuable services for the American people than that administered by the National Institutes of Health.[50]

Senator Hill in fact used the Woolridge Committee report as the major reason why the Senate should go along with the appropriations subcommittee's recommended increases, over the budget proposals, of $30 million. There were two additional arguments, both relating to persistent congressional interests and concerns. First, Hill reported to the Senate that while Congress had increased NIH funds substantially in the last 10 years, "the funds granted for medical research by private organizations have increased from $60 million a year to $600 million a year." The private and governmental sectors had both had a tenfold increase in their support. Second, Hill thought his colleagues would be interested to know what had been accomplished in recent years in heart research alone. "Surgeons operate and remove the aorta, the largest vessel in the body, and insert a plastic tube in its place. Dr. Miller, a former member of the

House, recently had 3½ feet of blood vessel taken out of his legs, and a plastic tube inserted. He is now healthy and normal." There was only one more thing. The chairman wanted to conclude by expressing his appreciation to the ranking Republican member of the subcommittee, Norris Cotton, the "distinguished Senator from New Hampshire, for his many fine contributions to this bill . . . I appreciate the fine work he did, and the fine help he gave not only to the subcommittee, but to the full committee." [51]

The Senator from New Hampshire was going along with the increases that year, although he did so grudgingly. He really thought things might be getting out of hand again, and he did want to raise "a red flag of warning, in a sense, for Senators to take notice in the future." But, he said,

> If we can afford to spend another $3 billion . . . in the foreign aid program around the world, if we can afford to build roads in Appalachia . . . contribute to paying the rents of some of our citizens, afford vast housing programs, if we can chase all the rainbows we are chasing as a national government—much of which I view with increasing apprehension and alarm—we would be in a poor position to take the time of the Senate fighting too long over a few million dollars added to the programs of research to prevent cancer, to seek a cure for cancer, to fight heart disease and respiratory diseases, and in support of all the other fine causes which are being carried on by the National Institutes of Health.[52]

There was no use fighting about the matter that year. Even Senator Proxmire, who usually introduced an amendment "to reduce the excess amount," decided that the cause was hopeless. It was an ironic situation, he suggested, because the Johnson Administration "has demonstrated over and over again that it has the deepest compassion for the health of the American people." Indeed, "future historians may well look back on the Johnson Administration as one of the greatest in history in its fervent interest in the health of Americans." But apparently because "what happened to Barry Goldwater last November seems to have paralyzed Republicans as well as Democrats," he found that he could not "get enough votes to put in your hat for this kind of amendment." So he would not only *not* introduce an amendment, he wouldn't even continue talking about the matter.[53] In one of the briefest discussions of the NIH appropriation bill in years, the Senate accepted on a voice vote the report of its appropriations subcommittee adding $30 million for NIH to what the House had voted.[54] And in the end, the final figure agreed upon by both houses was $896 million, $30 million more than the Johnson Administration had asked for. For fiscal 1967, Congress finally got the NIH budget over the one-billion-dollar mark by adding more than $64 million to the Administration request.

Bolstered by increased Democratic majorities in both houses (37 freshmen Democrats added to the House rolls) the ardent subcommittee chairmen, John Fogarty and Lister Hill, did not have to bargain with their Republican counterparts in 1965. More importantly, bolstered by an independent, outside report, the friends of medical research in Congress overcame an independent, inside attempt to retard the Cause. Simultaneously, Congress regained the initiative in promoting the medical research enterprise. The halcyon days had gone, but for the time being the congressional policy makers were back in dominant positions.

President Johnson was taking keener interest in medical research than his predecessors had. His friend Mary Lasker, who could see him any time she wished, was an important reason for that.[55] The President made speeches about medical research, visited the National Institutes of Health, praised the Woolridge Committee for its "excellent suggestions," and added $80 million to the NIH budget for 1966 over what it had been in 1965.

In an interview in the summer of 1965, Congressman Fogarty was asked whether he thought the President was trying to gain control over the medical research enterprise and lodge it securely in the executive branch. "Yes," was the reply, "but he'll never do it." [56]

He didn't do it that year, or the next year, in fiscal terms. But for fiscal 1968 the President's budget prevailed. One reason was that in January 1967, on the opening day of the Ninetieth Congress, John Fogarty died of a heart attack.

IX   The Breakdown of the Coalition

The triune force behind the medical research enterprise was the envy of some and the despair of others. Whether or not one approved of the means, or the ends, of the congressional-medical research agency-research lobby coalition, it seemed the perfect arrangement for the attainment of desired objectives.

For a good decade from the time that John Fogarty, Lister Hill, and James Shannon assumed their respective posts in 1954 and 1955, neither presidents, nor their cabinet secretaries in charge of health, nor their special offices for coordinating science policy could effectively control the direction or the pace of the federal biomedical research effort. Especially did officials whose jobs, according to organization charts, were the coordination of programs and control of budgets complain about the baronial league which took scant notice of the central administration's purposes, purse, or policy processes.

Senators who were unsuccessful in securing more funds for other causes wondered aloud what the secret weapon was that their colleague from Alabama had: one suggestion in reply was that it was a matter of personal charm, but another pointed to the powerful and ubiquitous lobby that supported and reinforced him in myriad ways.

Various commentators on the phenomenon varyingly emphasized the importance of individuals involved. The political good fortune of medical research, declared one, lay in the simple fact that one Senator and one Congressman, each a champion of the Cause, held key positions which enabled them to work their will on the rest of Congress and on the policy machinery of the government.[1] In occasional pieces written about her, and in the minds of some in government who remarked wonderingly on the matter, Mary Lasker was dubbed the single most important person behind the whole crusade to make medical research a foremost national cause.[2] Especially in the university world, including the numerous organizations in Washington representing particular segments of it, Dr. James Shannon was singled out for praise as the man who presided over the administration of the enterprise, reconciling needs and attitudes and expectations of policy makers on one side and of research performers on the other. Shannon was seen as the great welding force without whom the national medical research effort could not successfully endure.

Most observers recognized that it was the combination, the trifold alliance, that meant power. Describing it in personal rather than in group alliance terms, and emphasizing the sequential order of pertinent annual events, Elizabeth Brenner Drew summed up the outside view of the arrangement of the 1950's and 1960's: "in raising the [NIH] budget, Fogarty, Hill, Shannon and Lasker performed each year as a highly polished quartet." [3]

The image of alliance and quartets is oversimplified and can be misleading. In fact, there had never been a formal alliance with a definite charter. True, both the Senator from Alabama and the Congressman from Rhode Island had been influenced in the conduct of their responsibilities by Mrs. Lasker and her allies in the private sector; and their very important friend, Surgeon General Leonard Scheele, had picked Dr. Shannon for the NIH directorship. But the key members of Congress, research lobby leaders, and biomedical science bureaucrats had never sat down together and drawn up a set of goals or even a strategic plan for attaining goals presumably shared, implicitly agreed upon.

Mrs. Lasker was in Dr. Shannon's office only once, and spoke to him only a few times, in all the years they nonetheless worked in the same vineyard. Indeed, from an early if not precisely fixed point during the time when the informal coalition was shaping up, Mrs. Lasker and Dr. Shannon developed reservations about each other—reservations which produced the curious result that each readily courted every other potential friend of their common cause, but would not communicate with the other. It is important to remember, however, that although Mrs. Lasker was the founder and titular leader of the medical research lobby, she was not the whole thing; nor did other members of that interest group merely follow her lead or perform in public at her behest. If she did not communicate with Dr. Shannon, Mike Gorman, Sidney Farber, Michael DeBakey, and a host of others considered to be a part of the lobby certainly did. Besides, Mrs. Lasker was very keen about certain institute directors, and she did communicate with them.

There was at least a felt kinship in the early years between the lay and professional advocates outside government, the research-oriented members of Congress, and the agency officials. While Dr. Shannon had no intention of adopting the apparently passive stance of his predecessor, Dr. Sebrell, he nonetheless wanted to work in harness with his bureau's congressional and extragovernmental friends.

Like Surgeon General Scheele, Dr. Shannon appreciated the fact that friends in key places outside the executive branch could be as important in building a great enterprise as those within the executive. But Shannon also recognized that the combination of the lobby and the Congress could pose threats as well as offer support. Soon after assuming the directorship of NIH, he began making a quiet effort to strengthen the position of the bureau in the baronial league so as to reduce its vulnerability to the influence of outside forces, especially the medical research lobby. One way he did this was to get as close as possible to John Fogarty, with whom he fortunately shared an appreciation of a good drink.

In any case, there very definitely was a de facto coalition. And the success of its operational approach obscured some basic differences of view, differences which, ironically though not uniquely, became more pronounced as new boundaries were attained and new explorations christened. The nature of the coalition, meaning the nature of its members, produced, simultaneously with victories, increasing internal strains.

The differences among them reflected the styles and frames of reference of the persons and groups involved in the Cause, but they also represented different emphases about goals. And in the end, the differences became so significant that they resulted in a plain, old-fashioned power struggle. Yet, strangely, when the struggle became an open one it was not widely recognized as such; for two opposing forces were merely acting as seconds, each sending in a new principal to do battle—the President of the United States for the research lobby and the science community for the NIH directorate. Except for those who followed the politics of medical research closely, few recognized that the triune force had virtually come apart.

For Mary Lasker, her lay colleagues, and many of her doctor-scientist friends, the conquest of disease was not just a slogan to arouse popular support. It was a real cause, a crucial and obtainable goal. After all, Mrs. Lasker says, polio, tuberculosis, and most other diseases of bacteriological origin have largely been conquered. "I'm really opposed to heart attacks and cancer and strokes the way I'm opposed to sin," she has said.[4] Not that there was any question in any of the research advocates' minds about how disease was to be conquered; all knew it would take the development of a broad base of knowledge, the sophistication of scientific techniques, and the training of great numbers of additional scientific and medical personnel. But for Mrs. Lasker, once a relatively solid base was established the next moves should be bold ones. Every promising lead should be followed up vigorously, quickly, widely. Money should not be a deterrent; nor should the niceness of definition of a problem, the exquisiteness of scientific approach. Positing the goal—conquering cancer and other killer diseases—the outside professionals wanted to marshal every resource toward it as fast as possible.

The biomedical scientists, on the other hand, felt uncomfortable with a goal that was at once so specific and so grandiose. Of course finding answers to the affliction of disease was the ultimate hope. But there were more immediate problems to be attacked, and they had to be attacked carefully, systematically, step by step. The policy goals of the medical research enterprise that was being built therefore should not be stated in such dramatic terms. The basic problem of knowledge gaps must be the goal directly and immediately focused upon; more had to be discovered about genetics, biochemistry, molecular biology, biophysics, immunology. Then on to the next level of understanding, and the next and the next, in the biosciences. Subsequently, when the knowledge base was sufficient, when understanding of its critical components became finely honed, then a major, focused attack on specific diseases could be mounted with reasonable expectation of success. Meanwhile, it was also possible that a less differentiated approach to biomedical research might produce surprises with immediate relevance. Some of the most important medical breakthroughs, after all, had come from efforts in other fields than those being explored at the time.

The conquest of disease for the biomedical researcher was a result to be hoped for, but not a goal to be emblazoned on the laboratory door. "While scientists tend to view disease impersonally as a problem to be solved, Mrs. Lasker despises it —as she does all ugliness—considering it an enemy to be stamped out." [5] The NIH directorate, science trained and scientist oriented, usually came down on the side of the scientists.

No doubt Dr. James Shannon, director of the National Institutes of Health from 1955 to 1968—lush times for medical research—also wanted to find a cure for cancer and other "hazards to human life and health." But with scientific caution he rarely said so. To focus all available energies and resources so rigidly was to invite disappointment; unhappily, there simply was no "broad general theory, such as exists in the physical sciences," on which a massive assault on specific maladies could be solidly mounted. Thus, stated Dr. Shannon: "The development of diagnostic, therapeutic and preventive capability will continue to be dependent upon empirical approaches, serendipity, and the brilliance of too few gifted individuals." [6]

Targeted research, research aimed at finding cures for particular health problems, was in Dr. Shannon's view not only the most expensive but certainly the most chancy and not infrequently the most wasteful kind. The waste was not limited to dollars, but included use of scientific energies, for research efforts narrowly aimed at single targets could restrict beneficial effects of the internal dynamics of science. Moreover, for NIH to place too much emphasis on directed research would be to retard the development of science in another way: it could artificially skew the production of new biomedical scientists.

Shannon thought the first great goal of those pushing medical research as a major national endeavor should simply be the construction of biomedical science enterprise itself: the creation of a strong network of science-oriented universities and other institutions housing increasing numbers of researchers engaged in a "broad and free-ranging inquiry into all aspects of the phenomena of life, limited only by the criteria of excellence, intrinsic scientific importance, and the seriousness and competence of the investigator." To focus on more specific goals was to invite frustration, because given the present state of knowledge there were only "limited possibilities for highly organized research of a national nature with specific short-range goals." [7]

In the later years of his advocacy, John Fogarty was indignant at the notion that his and the Congress' only aim was the simplistic one of stamping out disease. He attacked the suggestion that the construction of an elaborate context for the attainment of the ultimate goal was something that occurred incidentally and outside of his purposeful design. Fogarty, Hill, Laird, and other congressional leaders came to know what a slow process and what a complex system were required before medical breakthroughs on a wide front would be achieved. They knew that whether or not disease was in fact being conquered, medical schools were being financially helped (at least for the short term) by medical research. It was mainly the congressional newcomers to the Cause who, in the first blush of their inevitable excitement, wondered why we didn't just pull all stops and go conquer cancer.[8]

Every year the experts of the House and Senate Appropriations Subcommittees explained to their colleagues the necessity of building up a base of knowledge, largely developed by scientists following their own leads, before it could be expected that disease could be ended. Senator Hill's report to the Senate in 1966 stated: "The committee continues to be convinced that progress of medical knowledge is basically dependent upon full support of undirected basic or applied research efforts of scientists working together or in groups." [9] The leaders continued their reminders that progress depended upon training new generations of scientific talent, and on insuring the fiscal and physical adequacy of science-performing institutions, in order to secure medical advances.

Every year also, the committees insisted that the directors of the component institutes of NIH and the citizen witnesses concerned with specific diseases put on record evidences of specific problems and specific progress. More cautious than the lobbyists who pulled them from one side, and more daring than the science administrators who held back on the other, congressional leaders simultaneously goaded the research agency to undertake new, sizable developmental efforts and refrained from interfering in the Shannon plan to build, broaden, and reinforce the basic structure. And every year, side by side with the paragraphs stating the case for basic research in the formal committee report, and in the oral report to the respective houses of Congress, the leaders and their friends cited examples both of medical progress and of personal tragedies because there had not been greater progress, to insure acceptance of their proposed increases for medical research. If there were those skeptical of their scientific, organizational, or economic logic, perhaps an emotional appeal might persuade.

Lyndon B. Johnson as Senate Majority Leader rose to support Senator Hill's plea for more money for medical research, and especially for cancer, in June 1959. The committee had compiled impressive statistics to document its case that progress had been made and more could be expected; but Senator Johnson reminded, "while we are beginning to achieve remarkable breakthroughs against cancer, it still kills 225,000 Americans every year." Not only that, "over the last decade alone cancer has claimed the lives of five members of this body [including] . . . the beloved Matt Neely, who by a bitter twist of fate died of the disease which he had been fighting legislatively for more than 20 years." Johnson hoped and prayed that as a result of the vision and the efforts of Senator Hill and his co-workers in the Cause "the day will come when we drive from the face of the earth these dread diseases which cost so much in pain and suffering and money each year we live." [10]

Support from some colleagues related more to a collegial spirit, to norms of committee unity and personal friendship and mutual backscratching, than to convictions on what the medical research enterprise was, could be, or should do. But a critical if numerically indeterminate bloc of support came from those who wanted to conquer disease and who believed that conquest was assured if not imminent. Ben Jensen's hopes, fears, and goals were as basic as his help was critical. His attitude is revealed in this query of a physician witness who appeared before the House subcommittee: "Doctor, I have been greatly interested in your testimony. I want to say right now on the record that I thank God we have men like you and the rest of those folks who are schooled in the art of medicine and surgery for suffering humanity. Is cancer prevalent among people who work out of doors, like farmers?" [11]

Even more revealing, and more important an indication of goals held by the legislative members of the tripartite alliance for the advancement of medical research, was the fact that it was Congress that had decided upon the categorical disease approach in the first instance and Congress that had continued to insist upon it.

Congress agreed in 1950 to leave principal initiative to the Surgeon General for creating new insititutes when he thought it desirable.[12] On such initiative, several new institutes were created. Meanwhile, congressional interest in naming institutes after specific health problems never waned. Aside from urging the creation of some of the new institutes and insisting on others (for example, the National Eye Institute), Congress prodded NIH and the Surgeon General to rename the Microbiology Institute, which involved one of the oldest activities of the agency, so as to make its function better understood and its mission more salable. ("Whoever died of microbiology?" asked one knowing wag.[13]) In 1955 it became the National Institute of Allergy and Infectious Diseases.

In sum, regardless of the sophistication of key members of Congress about the nature of the research enterprise—their recognition of the essentiality of having solid underpinnings of basic knowledge, of giving individual scientists free reign, of the need for and possibilities of indirection and serendipity in research—the basic goals of Congress seemed clear. True, they were engaged in selling less sophisticated colleagues on their plan and in encouraging public support, and perhaps they had to simplify matters somewhat. But what they had in mind was really quite precise. The purpose of the categorical disease institutes and the goal of national medical research policy was "to improve the health of the people of the United States through the conduct of researches, investigations, experiments, and demonstrations relating to cause, prevention, and method of diagnosis and treatment of diseases." [14]

At the crossroads of national decision after World War II, the National Institutes of Health had critical need of strong congressional friends and a powerful citizen clientele. Otherwise it could have gotten lost in the shuffle of research contracts and policy alternatives and proposed new organizations and research emphases. Had it not been for the combination of an understandable, extended national debate about the government's postwar research policy with the unpredictable emergence of a congressional-citizen alliance which decided to champion NIH as the nation's major medical research arm, that bureau of the Public Health Service might well have been doomed to a limited, gradually withering role.

Under such circumstances, the agency could not help but yield to its friends' emphasis on disease problems and solutions rather than continue in its historic preference for the exploration of basic science, its self-determined research goals. Surgeon General Thomas Parran thought the time was right for an attack on disease, but others more closely tied to the laboratory balked. A sort of modus vivendi was worked out by Dr. C. J. Van Slyke, whose ground rules accommodated, superficially at least, all parties: in any "attack" on disease, the researcher was to be as free as possible of red tape and was to be free to follow his own leads. And if some thought the charge to the agency given by the statutory fathers, "to improve the health of the people of the United States" by focusing on one disease at a time, was too restrictive, Dr. Van Slyke suggested that it was actually a very broad mandate. "Hell," he said, "we can support anything —the whole body is bathed in blood." [15]

In the early years of its operation, each group in the coalition —lobbyists, members of Congress, research agency officials— approached the operation diplomatically, gingerly. Each had its natural proclivities and preferences, some recognizable early on. But what was clearer to each than potential divergence of view was present mutual need. It took several years of participation on advisory councils for the outside professionals to get a sufficient "feel" of NIH before they were prepared to challenge its management on particular emphases and approaches. It took congressional leaders a few years to decide that they could successfully persuade their colleagues to accelerate the expenditure of public monies for medical research, and successfully pressure the research agency to accelerate its pace and the expansion of its program range. For its part, gratified as it was for the lobby's and the Congress' support, NIH would accommodate the other coalition members' desires so far as it could. Thus were the differences muted.

As time went on, the interested extragovernmental supporter, whether layman or medical professional, moved from general exhortations (to the advisory councils, the NIH directorate, and the Congress) on moving faster toward solving health problems by spending more money, to more specific efforts to effectuate more specific research possibilities. The first step was usually to take the matter up directly with the institute director, or perhaps the director of NIH. Another approach, complementary or alternative, was to sell the pertinent advisory council on the proposal. Failing receipt of cooperation by the institutes, the outside professional might go directly to Senator Hill or Congressman Fogarty and get him to intercede with the NIH directorate. Indeed, many of the early struggles between research lobbyists and NIH management were played out quietly behind the scenes in the offices of Hill or Fogarty. If attracted to an idea proposed by Mrs. Lasker or Dr. Farber or another friend, Hill might invite Dr. Shannon down to discuss the proposition. If Shannon had reservations, Hill usually respected them and urged Shannon to come up with an alternative plan that would move in the direction desired by the outside professional, but not necessarily exclusively involving the proposed researcher or the same scale of operation. Occasionally Hill was insistent, and Shannon might, if he felt strongly about the matter, then turn to Fogarty to get him involved on the other side. Generally speaking, Mrs. Lasker, Mrs. Mahoney, Dr. Farber, and Dr. DeBakey turned a little more readily to Senator Hill to get their pet projects launched, and Dr. Shannon turned a little more readily to his fellow Irishman John Fogarty. But the situation was sometimes reversed, and in any case was flexible.

Usually an accommodation could be worked out, but whether or not it was (whether in fact the idea for a new project or new research direction originated in the same informal way from scientist-administrators at NIH), the language of the congressional committee reports frequently caused them to read like unilateral directives to NIH.

Sometimes the directives were general: "The Committee is quite dissatisfied with the overall progress made by this institute. It is the oldest institute and, with a single exception has consistently received the highest level of support . . . It is of very substantial consequence to the Committee, and to the American people generally, that we set the stage for some real progress." [16] Or, "the Committee is surprised to find that there is such a dearth of research in the field of hemophilia. This is certainly not in keeping with the magnitude of the problem. The Committee will expect that a portion of the increase be used to strengthen this research." [17]

Occasionally the commands were a little more explicit: "The committee directs the National Institutes of Health to establish training programs designed to draw into the field of medical research, broadly defined, scientists of high competence in specialized areas of chemistry and physics." [18] Or, "the Committee will expect that clinical drug trials be continued and expanded." [19]

Dr. Shannon maintained as late as 1965 that the congressional committees had never pushed him to engage in a research effort that he objected to. Congress, he said, despite its understandable zeal and desire for practical results, had been quite reasonable on this score. He suggested that what appeared to be congressional directives to the agency were in fact directives that NIH had approved in advance if not originated.[20] Colleagues of Shannon believe that is too sweeping a statement and admit that some programs—cystic fibrosis, retrolental fibroplasia, cancer chemotherapy among others—were more the children of Congress than of NIH. Shannon's willingness to accommodate the citizens' lobby and the congressional committees in earlier years was apparently matched by an unwillingness to admit that anyone other than himself and his associates had control over the research enterprise. Even when the lobby, through Mike Gorman and Dr. Nathan Kline, launched a public attack on the director of the National Institute of Mental Health, Dr. Shannon played down the implications of stress within the coalition offered by the example. He thought, he said, that the institute director had been overly conservative, unnecessarily reluctant in moving forward with the psychopharmacological program which the National Committee Against Mental Illness was so keen on; what they thought was the Mental Health Institute's purposeful stymying of the program had prompted their outburst against the director in the congressional hearings.

But Shannon himself began to feel the pressure of the outside professionals. They employed a public forum to attack his "conservatism" in 1962 on a similar problem.

The background was that in 1961 a directive was placed in the Senate report urging NIH to proceed with the development of "categorical clinical research centers, specifically oriented toward major disease areas such as cancer, cardiovascular diseases, mental health, and neurological diseases." The Committee specifically directed that "the sums appropriated for strengthening clinical research resources will be used only for this purpose." [21]

Shannon was increasingly bothered by the categorical approach to research and increasingly vocal in his opposition. Besides his continuing feelings about the undesirable skewing of manpower and the uncertainty that such category specifications really help obtain categorical results, he was under increasing pressure from grantee institutions who were finding the expanding numbers of categorical research awards particularly frustrating: they caused unnatural divisions of labor, extra red tape, and in some cases disruption of internally decided personnel and program balances. For such reasons, Shannon preferred a multicategorical approach.

Congress reflected on its past experience and its continuing need to sell medical research in hard, understandable terms and pushed for the categorical clinics. In a diverting move, Shannon used a directive of the Secretary of Health, Education and Welfare to all bureaus of the Department to reduce their budgets by taking the necessary cuts out of the clinical research programs. Mike Gorman, among others, was upset, and he tried mightily to stir up the anger of the House committee.

> Over the past three years both House and Senate reports have clearly indicated that they wanted NIH to develop clinical research centers in various regions of the country to direct their attacks upon specific diseases.
>
> However, the Director of the National Institutes of Health, who is enamored of the so-called multicategorical approach—which presumably covers everything from the 1-day cold to the 7-year itch—has chosen to misunderstand for reasons of his own.
>
> I respect him greatly, but he has chosen, I think, to misunderstand in this case clear congressional directive. However, he is not fuzzy when it comes to cutting money from a program. When Secretary Ribicoff ordered a $60 million cut in the fiscal 1962 NIH budget—that is, the overall cut—the Director of the National Institutes of Health pounced on the $31 million voted by the Congress, by the House and the Senate, for the categorical clinical research centers and reduced them by a whopping $15 million—that is, from $31 million to $16 million.
>
> I think a lot of blood hit the floor at that point. He did

not, Mr. Chairman—I must emphasize—take one dollar from his precious multicategorical amorphous, metabolic, or whatever program centers.[22]

However the agency may have chafed under such pressure, it was not Congress that bore the brunt of its unhappiness. Congress, after all, was still the most important reason for its healthy condition; it would not snap at the hand that had fed it in its lean days even if it was getting a little choosier about menu selections and portion sizes. As far as Director Shannon was concerned, his was not an entirely unhappy position.

Not that it was an ideal situation, mind you. What would have been preferable, suggested Dr. Shannon, was to have the executive branch of government make a genuine, comprehensive assessment of needs and possibilities and commit itself to a realistic and progressive program of health research. He put the story to the Fountain Committee in 1962 as follows:

I might say that we have had only two opportunities while I have held an administrative position in the National Institutes of Health to attempt to define our need and opportunity in terms of reasonable budgets.

Traditionally, from about 1950, when I first took part in this, the budget submission has reflected the expenditures characteristic of the then current year rather than any attempt of the executive branch to develop a profound assessment.

I think this is bad in two ways. It really relegates to the Congress the total leadership in the defining of program areas and their rate of development; and for the operating agency it means that its planning is always after the fact of the budget accomplishment rather than before it.

Our present difficulties are not a result of the rapid increase itself, but of the mechanism by which this rapid rate has come about—where the Congress has had to take charge. And I don't blame them for that, for goodness knows the need is there.

But I do blame the executive branch for its refusal to be responsive to the very broad social drive in this Nation toward better health. The only opportunity to obtain that better health is through research. This is well perceived . . . The unwillingness or inability of the executive branch to acknowledge this drive has led consistently—except for one year—to a failure to permit realistic budgeting for these programs, from serious planning to the actual appropriation.[23]

Absent such concern and interest on the part of the executive branch, Dr. Shannon simply did the best he could to live with what he considered to be the unrealistic budgets he was permitted to submit to Congress, the pressures accompanying the support of outside interest groups, the short planning time frame allowed under the circumstances, the needs and demands of the grantee institutions and the scientific community, the pushing of the appropriations subcommittees and now the pulling of the Fountain Committee. Actually, he did very well indeed. So well, in fact, that he tacitly acknowledged that it was he who ran NIH, who made all the critical decisions about where the agency would go and how fast, and no one else. Congress was by and large "very thoughtful and very considerate." [24] And (up to 1965 anyway) the outside professionals were actually quite helpful and not dysfunctional or irresponsible. Not ideal, his situation, but he was coping rather nicely.

There were other perspectives about why the enterprise was achieving a reputation for success and why its function, the performance of medical research designed to reduce physical affliction, continued to receive strong public support. One such perspective was that it was because the agency's political sponsors, on whom it depended for the continuing largesse of public expenditures showered upon it, kept the agency's focus and energies in part on practical results.

Prompted by a curious mixture of scientific and political success on the one hand and lack of greater success in producing specific disease cures on the other, the outside professionals began to push the professional scientific managers ever harder. The NIH directorate had been reluctant, in the mid-fifties, to embark on a wide-ranging program of clinically testing chemical agents against cancer. Based on analyses presented by trusted friends like Dr. Sidney Farber, Congress believed chemotherapy to hold great promise, and it provided ever greater amounts of money for the cancer chemotherapy program. In proposing $24 million above the House recommendation for the National Cancer Institute in 1960, the Senate Appropriations Subcommittee indicated that the chemotherapy program was one area where it wished to see increased activity. "The committee . . . directs that expansion of clinical investigation proceed as rapidly as the clinical and scientific resources of the country permit." [25]

The results of the endeavor were mixed: by the early sixties chemotherapy had proved to be a significant advance in cancer treatment; but the scientific advance came despite managerial and other organizational problems. Those problems led one of the several committees assessing various aspects of the NIH operation to recommend that no similar programs be undertaken in the future, regardless of scientific merit, before an adequate management team could be assembled.[26]

Congressional friends of NIH, at any rate, thought the cancer chemotherapy program successful. "It seems clear," stated the House committee report for fiscal 1960, "that the last five years of tooling up for this gigantic program are now paying off." [27]

A few years earlier there had been similar promise in a chemotherapeutic approach to mental illness, but NIH held back, believing that a major program of clinical testing in the field would be premature. Similarly, the NIH directorate continued to resist moving ahead in cancer chemotherapy. Timing was always extremely important, and the time was not yet right.

It seemed to outside professionals that the NIH directorate had lapsed into a mentality typified by the old Hygienic Laboratory's microbiologists. Somehow the timing never seemed quite right, to Dr. Shannon, for the exploitation of a recently uncovered possibility. And his constant emphasis on the importance of basic research, his disapproval of any further "disease category" approach to research, his opposition to clinical centers, were perceived as a pattern or posture indicating less than a burning zeal to get promising research results—likely medical relief—to real people, to suffering individuals who needed help.

It was recognized that Dr. Shannon's judgment in many of these matters reflected that of working scientists themselves. The researchers were unquestionably the experts on microscientific factors; and they were of course well motivated. The problem, said Mrs. Lasker, was that "too many of them are without a deep sense of urgency." Said Mike Gorman: "We figure they get the seven-year itch in about eight years." [28]

Such lay opinion was shared by some of the doctor-scientists among the outside professionals. Dr. Farber argues that it is not necessary to have absolutely complete and pure understanding of every factor of a given agent which has been demonstrated to be effective, before applying it toward the reduction of pain and illness. He points out that medical scientists still do not totally understand the "mechanism of action" of aspirin, insulin, or antihypertension drugs.[29]

Dr. Howard Rusk would agree. He lost a battle with "AMA types and research purists" in the early fifties when he proposed supplying isoniazid tablets on a massive scale in Korea to try to check the near-epidemic level of tuberculosis (2.5 million cases out of a population of 15 million) because those opposing him argued that the drug had not been sufficiently tested. It was subsequently accepted as a most efficacious agent, and Dr.

Rusk still thinks he was right in recommending its use before every shadow of doubt was cleared up. His position is that in cases of desperate need and proportions, typical and ordinarily admirable scientific caution, which seeks perfection of means as well as ends, should give way to bold experimentation.[30]

Dr. Shannon blocked Dr. DeBakey's efforts to have NIH support the development of an artificial heart in 1966 because he thought it would be premature. To make his point about premature development in medicine, he volunteered an opinion that the National Foundation had erred, years earlier, in releasing the Salk polio vaccine at a time when a much improved vaccine was forthcoming. The Foundation responded by reminding Shannon that the Salk vaccine was in use, and saving lives, five years before the Sabin formula was ready for distribution.[31]

The *New York Times* entered this fray. In an editorial it said: "In reviving this controversy, Dr. Shannon comes close to saying that it is a mistake to act until almost total knowledge is available. But is this perfectionist position justified? Edward Jenner did not possess enough basic knowledge when he did so much to introduce smallpox vaccination more than a century and a half ago. By modern standards, he was a simpleton who did not even know the germ theory of disease, let alone the viral origin of smallpox." [32]

Congress' natural and persistent desire for practical results was said to be the reason for its frequently siding with the outside professionals against the research agency's directorate. No doubt that was one consideration; its own experience in seeing positive results from some of its own initiatives—cervical cancer mass testing and beginning cystic fibrosis, rubella, and deafness research programs—suggested that it could be done. But aside from what were nonetheless potentially unrealistic expectations causing Congress to push NIH into the new fields of endeavor, congressional leaders in the medical research cause had come to recognize the usual inherent caution of the scientific mind. And while that cautious approach was thoroughly respected by Congress, what had also become familiar was the value of the exception to that approach. The story of a medical breakthrough despite peer skepticism which Dr. Irving Wright told Senator Hill in 1956 was one the likes of which Hill had heard before and would hear again and again.

> Dr. Wright: We therefore started to treat a series of patients suffering from coronary thrombosis with anticoagulate therapy. This was in 1942.
> Senator Hill: That was pioneering, so to speak.
> Wright: That is right. And it was looked on by us as a pilot study.
> Hill: And I suppose you met great resistance, did you not?
> Wright: Great resistance.
> Hill: That is the usual story, is it not?
> Wright: At first [they say] "it couldn't be so," and later, "we knew it all the time." [33]

As the medical research coalition members came to recognize the fact of their collective political success, it produced a curious effect upon them separately. They began to be more assertive against each other. The NIH directorate was less and less inclined to do the bidding of the Congress or the outside professionals unless that bidding was in accord with NIH aims. The medical science bureaucrats developed strategies of getting around even relatively specific congressional directives, as the Gorman attack on Shannon indicates. The Congress, more comfortable and more sophisticated now, used the outside professionals for their own purposes more and more. The citizen witnesses' testimony was reportedly considered as "window dressing" by Congressman Fogarty; what he claimed to go by was the "professional judgments" of the individual institute directors.[34]

For their part, the outside professionals and laymen, having established an influential position over the research budget, now began focusing more attention on the substance of the program. Their greatest and most obvious success had been the creation of heart, cancer, and stroke centers in major medical centers around the country. Beginning with a plank in the Democratic platform in 1960 which called for the creation of a presidential commission to study the matter, then persuading two presidents subsequently of the importance of the idea, next having Dr. DeBakey named chairman when the committee was appointed by President Johnson in the spring of 1964 —the outside professionals next saw the recommendations they made six months later become law in record time. They had lost a year's time due to President Kennedy's assassination; but by 1965 their concept of a national network of facilities, focusing on the indicated diseases and combining research, training, and patient care, had become a statutory fact.[35] They believed the next thrust of the enterprise should consist of wide-scale field trials of drugs, large collaborative research efforts, and new combinations of research-clinical testing centers.

Part of the medical research lobby also continued to push the cancer chemotherapy program. Having gotten money committed to the effort, the next step was to insure that it was spent properly. From 1960 to 1965, the outside professionals and Congress on one side and the NIH directorate on the other waged a symptomatic tug-of-war over the matter of research contracts on cancer chemotherapy. The National Advisory Cancer Council, on which Dr. Farber and Mrs. Lasker were serving in 1963, asked to review proposals invited by the Cancer Institute and submitted by interested industrial laboratories. The NIH directors balked. There was nothing in the statute giving advisory councils review authority over contracts—merely over grants. Council members thought this ludicrous; their role was to oversee the whole research effort in the cancer field, especially that performed outside NIH but supported by it. Mrs. Lasker and Dr. Farber took the matter to their friends on Capitol Hill; the Senate and House Appropriations Subcommittees issued instructions, through their reports, that the Council was to review contracts as well as grants. In the words of the Senate report on proposed appropriations for fiscal 1964: "All moneys allocated in this contractual program shall be spent only after review by the National Advisory Cancer Council." [36]

As Dr. Shannon and his colleagues saw it, the Council seemed to be asking for control over the internal operations of the Cancer Institute. He appealed to the Secretary of Health, Education and Welfare, John W. Gardner, for support. Secretary Gardner backed NIH, and asked the Senate and House committees not to press the matter before he could have a study made of the policy issues involved. Hill and Fogarty agreed, and Gardner appointed an eight-man committee chaired by Dr. Jack Ruina, president of the Institute for Defense Analysis, a Pentagon-supported think-tank.[37] The committee supported the Shannon-Gardner position against the contract review authority claimed by the Council.[38]

Secretary Gardner's intervention on behalf of the NIH directorate signaled several new factors. First, Dr. Shannon had come to be recognized as a major, independent figure in the medical research alliance and in the research enterprise. Important from the early days of his tenure, he had by 1964 built such a reputation in the biomedical science-university world that he was considered by many to be indispensable in the job. The fact that he had indicated he might resign if the contract review issue were not resolved in his favor was an important consideration in Gardner's intervention.

Second, the Secretary's putting himself at the center of responsibility over a medical research policy issue represented the first occasion since Marion Folsom's days on which the parent department of the research agency took a lively interest in critical matters. If it strengthened Shannon's hand vis-à-vis the Congress and the outside professionals, it also strengthened his dependence on Departmental leadership, without which he had operated for so long.

Aside from being one more indication that the executive generally was re-entering the premises, the Gardner intervention at Shannon's request signaled the escalation of the tensions among the policy triumvirate that had been controlling, virtually exclusively, national medical research policy.

Dr. Shannon naturally was pleased with the outcome of the issue. And he was particularly pleased that, after a long interval, he had the personal and organizational backing of the Secretary of HEW. Henceforth, in Shannon's mind, John Gardner would join Marion Folsom as one of the truly important reasons for what he considered was the success of the National Institutes of Health.[39] In a sense, he felt liberated from the Congress and the lobby who, ironically until the present, had been virtually his only political friends. As he told the Fountain Committee in 1962, although he appreciated those friends, the absence of real and realistic support from the executive branch made trying to run an executive agency and a national enterprise a rather difficult job.[40]

Presumably Dr. Shannon realized that Mrs. Lasker might also repair to the executive for additional support of her point of view in the developing struggle. She had, after all, been a friend of Lyndon Johnson since his days as Senate majority leader, and Lady Bird had twice visited her at her house in France on the Côte d'Azur. Johnson's first important support of the Cause came in 1959 when he made a speech (written by Mike Gorman) in support of the Senate Appropriations Subcommittee's request for an additional several million for the institutes. In 1961 as Vice President, he addressed the Lasker Awards luncheon. In 1965, Mrs. Lasker gave the First Lady an enormous boost with her beautification efforts, an area of keen mutual interest. Presidential aid Douglass Cater reported that when the President was preparing for surgery in 1965, Mary Lasker was the last person to see him before he left the White House for the hospital.[41]

Continuing to be impatient with NIH leadership, Mrs. Lasker decided it would take a presidential shove to move the agency and the researchers it supported out beyond their laboratorial fascinations. Of course basic research was essential; but after 10 years and $8-plus billion spent in building a great scientific base, surely the time had come for a special new thrust to get results to the victims of the diseases which, according to their statutory charges, the institutes of the NIH were supposed to be concerned with.[42]

On June 27, 1966, President Johnson invited the directors of the Institutes of Health, along with the Surgeon General of the Public Health Service and Secretary Gardner, to the White House for a discussion of how to get research results transformed into practical answers to disease problems. Calling the assembled group his "strategy council in the war against disease," the President asked whether "too much energy was being spent on basic research and not enough on translating laboratory findings into tangible benefits for the American people." [43] The President asked the NIH directorate to review priorities and if necessary to reshape them in order to get maximum results from existing programs.

The President's questions and requests were not unreasonable. But having been given no advance notice of what his concerns were, and being keenly aware of Mrs. Lasker's influence with him, the President's words fell like a bombshell on NIH officials. They were shaken, and so were their friends to whom the word was quickly passed. "The President's initiative . . . caused an explosion among the scientists and in the universities. They took it to mean that the Lasker forces were in the saddle; that support for applied research and development was to be substituted for support for basic research by an anti-intellectual, unsophisticated President who could never understand such things." [44]

Whatever else the President's initiative accomplished, it aroused the longtime, quietly demanding, ever-expecting major constituent and principal beneficiary of the National Institutes of Health—the universities—to vigorous if haphazard action. For the first time, academic administrators and scientists came forward in strong and unified ranks to enter the medical research policy arena. Rarely had institutional researchers or administrators asked or been asked to appear in the annual congressional sequence where fund levels were decided and new program initiatives often made, to underscore the need for basic research or caution against overemphasis on the immediately practical. In the course of occasional testimony by a medical school official, some brief comment was offered: "it is generally conceded that this support has been broadly conceived, rather than dedicated to narrowly categorized disease";[45] otherwise, the defense of priorities as favored by NIH and the grant recipients had been left to Dr. Shannon. Now the hitherto quiet beneficiaries began to yell, and the impact of their aggregate reaction effectively countered what they viewed as the illogical, irrational approach of the medical research lobby.

Concern was so widespread that Secretary Gardner made an effort to allay the fears and otherwise clear the heads of the science-university community by convoking a meeting with all NIH consultants in August to clarify the position of the Department and, implicitly, of the President. He told them, first, that there was to be no change in the policy of supporting fundamental research. He asked them to accept the fact that there was not a "fixed federal health dollar" for which basic research, applied and developmental efforts, and delivery of services had to compete, pointing out that the federal government was probably going to spend an ever larger share of its revenues on health generally. He reassured at least those whose concern was for the university as a whole more than for the individual scientist by suggesting that such new programs as the heart, cancer, and stroke centers and the regional medical programs would mean that "the future of one or another form of university extension activity in the medical field is going to be very lively indeed." [46] In short, whatever mix of federal health funds was decided upon in the future, the universities would continue to get theirs.

John Gardner's message, promptly transmitted to the affected community by its favorite "house organ," *Science*, was somewhat reassuring. And the President was possibly reassured by the subsequent report from the National Institutes of Health which claimed that 60 percent of its monies already went for "applied research" and specified items of medical progress resulting from medical research over the last two decades. The tentativeness of such reassurances was forgotten when the President helicoptered out to the Bethesda campus of the research enterprise in 1967 to laud the NIH directorate, staff, and grantees for their "billion dollar success story." [47] With that, the relations between the President and the science-university community achieved a condition of status quo ante bellum.

Douglass Cater, the special assistant to Lyndon Johnson who was the most frequent point of access to the President for both the Laskerites and the Shannonites, thought the struggle between the opposing points of view had aspects of "creative tension" out of which presumably came clearer choices, more purposeful endeavors.[48]

That assessment of the incident fits with the historical pattern of relationships between the politician and the science spokesman in the biomedical research field. But the most immediate, if not the most obvious, implication of the presidential challenge of 1966 and presidential reassurance of 1967 was that the old de facto research coalition had come apart. The war against disease gave way to open war among the troops.

X   The End of an Era

Perhaps it is inevitable that the cause of sustaining medical research as a top national priority seemed to run out of steam in the latter 1960's. A 10-year period of enthusiasm or even strong majority acceptance is usually as much as any great national plan can hope for before major troubles develop. Various national programs, from the Marshall Plan to the space effort, seem to have operated for about a decade in lush if not unthreatened environments before they fell on hard times, before other causes were perceived to have surpassed them in public importance, before avowed enemies or critically placed skeptics arose to pose damaging challenges, and their budgets began to level off or decline.

That the national medical research enterprise, as embodied in the activities of the National Institutes of Health, came so far so fast before serious troubles obscured its future is all the more impressive in that, for much of its life, it lacked high-priority treatment from the executive branch of government. Its growth began before 1955 and lasted beyond 1965, but during that decade, the strong, resilient coalition that directed it overcame every hurdle that stood in the way, including the occasional opposition of the Bureau of the Budget speaking for the President.

Trouble within the coalition came at a particularly unfortunate time, for the environment in which it had to operate had become more difficult, if not more hostile. A major factor in the climatic change was that research and development, whose importance had been born of the experience of war and buoyed by the continuance of the cold war and of space rivalry, gradually declined in popularity. The boom period for research and development had begun to level off by the mid-sixties, with congressional committees investigating federal research and development programs to determine, for one thing, whether there was "unnecessary waste and duplication," and for another, what the results were from the annual expenditure of $16 billion by the federal government for research and development.[1] In response to the latter question, the National Aeronautics and Space Administration, whose total budget was placed in the category of "R & D expenditures," could easily point with pride to great achievements in space, but it had to struggle to produce evidence that results of space research had also produced transferrable advantages for daily earthly activities. The Defense Department's "Project Hindsight," analyzing a spectrum of basic and otherwise nontargeted research efforts supported by the Department, revealed that there had been minimal results for practical nonmilitary purposes.

William D. Carey, executive assistant director of the Bureau of the Budget, had warned as early as in 1964 that a budget squeeze for research and development was in the making. In that year federal expenditures for research and development had topped $14.5 billion, and an exuberant aggregation of performers of federally sponsored research seemed to see no end to the growth curve of their major source of funds. Carey cautioned against such delusions about the attainment of the millennium, against the "state of mind that assumes that the miracle of the loaves and the fishes will go on indefinitely and that the mere assertion of a valid scientific need will suffice to turn on the financial gusher once more." He raised a specific caution: "I should like to make it very plain that the justification for the 16th and 17th billion [for all federal research and development programs] will have to be very different from the justification which sufficed for the first billion."[2] In the same year Dr. Charles V. Kidd, who had long been involved in central planning activities and in training programs of NIH added a special footnote for the biomedical sciences: a slowdown could be expected in that sector as well.[3]

A year or so earlier, however, other knowledgeable authorities on the government-university science arrangement—Alan Waterman, director of the National Science Foundation; Frederick Seitz, president of the National Academy of Sciences; Philip Handler, frequent panelist and adviser to government granting agencies (who later became president of the National Academy)—saw no reduction of the growth curve for search and development funds.[4] In 1962, when he was sitting on top of his happy empire, Dr. James Shannon predicted that the total national expenditure for biomedical research (then at the level of $1.3 billion from all sources) would reach $3 billion annually by 1970.[5] The dramatic (some would say traumatic) happenings of the last few years of the decade are suggested by the fact that the figure attained by 1970 was more than a half-billion dollars short of that. Actually, the $2 billion level was reached in 1966, and the increases since then have hardly kept pace with the rate of inflation.

It is clear that the national climate was conducive to research growth from 1950 to 1966, and that the public felt particularly strongly about funds for medical research. No doubt the national medical research enterprise would have grown without the ubiquitous, singleminded group of citizen boosters symbolized by Mary Lasker and their smooth, successful relationship with key members of Congress and the NIH directorate. But it is one indication of the potency of the coalition that while the total national expenditures for all research and development increased at an average annual rate of 14 percent between 1950 and 1960, funds for medical research increased at an annual rate of 17 percent for the same years. If the comparable growth curves are examined for the decade 1955–1965, when the medical research lobby was at its zenith, the difference is even greater. As for federal spending for "R & D" in that period, medical research is the only research activity that grew at a noticeably steeper rate than the budget makers of the executive branch wanted or planned.

There was, of course, a "negative factor" that must be added to the positive factor of zealous intelligence by the coalition in producing greater medical research budgets in those years. Along with public health programs and facilities construction programs, research remained one of few areas in which a congressman could cast a vote for health. Other avenues—health insurance, hospital care for the aged and indigent, federal aid to medical education—were blocked by a clearly self-serving lobby which was by many leagues more powerful, and which more brazenly fed popular fears, than anything the medical research lobby could hope to be or do. "Medical research," remarked Congressman Laird as he made ready to help boost its budget one more time, "is the best kind of health insurance" the American people could have.[6]

But the 1960's, and especially the elections of 1964, opened up new ways for the federal government to help improve and extend citizen health. In 1963, the Congress took a small but direct step toward federal aid for medical and paramedical education in passing the Health Professions Education Act, making possible grants and loans to schools training health personnel.[7] In 1965, Congress and the Administration finally broke the stranglehold the American Medical Association had on *any* plan to provide federally underwritten health insurance for any group of Americans, by enacting Medicare—providing hospital insurance for elderly recipients of social security—and Medicaid [8]—providing federal funds for state programs to cover the cost of certain medical care for the poor and the "medically indigent."

In the preceding decade, without those important and costly programs, medical research had risen from a figure comprising 30 percent of the total cost of all health programs of the Department of Health, Education and Welfare ($81 million out of a total of $288 million) to 37 percent in 1965 ($947 million out of a total of $2.571 billion). By 1970, the medical research component of the HEW budget had passed a billion dollars; but with Medicare and Medicaid on the books, the total HEW budget had jumped to more than $15.8 billion, with over $12 billion of that for Medicare and Medicaid.

Medical research, the health darling of the Department in earlier years, by the end of the decade represented only about 6 percent of HEW's health dollars. Medical research still was, despite controversies, less controversial than other health programs, but it was no longer the only standard by which to judge whether a congressman was "for health."

There was yet another ominous new factor for federal medical research budgets which was changing the environment: the cost of the war in Southeast Asia. President Johnson wanted and planned to increase expenditures of public monies on federal health and education programs, including new ones launched during his years in office, and he did so. As the cost of American military intervention in Vietnam increased (dramatically, with the giant step the President took into the war in 1965), the expectation was that domestic spending would suffer. Indeed it did in the last years of the decade, but not because the President did not try mightily to invalidate the historic rule that nations cannot have simultaneously adequate supplies of guns and butter to meet all needs. He could not stir Congress or the people to provide additional tax revenues that would be required to wage equally vigorous battle against "Communist aggressors" in Indochina and against a wide array of serious domestic ills, some only recently identified. In the end, the President who cared passionately about the people's health had to resort to the ways of some of his predecessors to keep the federal budget relatively intact: he placed restrictions on spending (on those programs he could) regardless of dollar amounts appropriated.

In the fiscal years 1967, 1968, and 1969, the last years of the Johnson presidency, Congress sequentially raised (1967), accepted (1968), and lowered (1969) the medical research agency's budget. But in each of those years, under strictures from the White House, NIH declined to spend sizable amounts of the money appropriated. Presidents Eisenhower and Kennedy had also put ceilings on spending when they thought the Congress had gone too far in "force-feeding" medical research. Further, the NIH directorate often turned some dollars back to the Treasury when it did not believe the money could be efficaciously spent, and its patrons in Congress approved. Dr. Shannon told the Fountain Committee that one of the reasons he thought Congress was so generous with the agency was that the subcommittee appropriations members knew no money would be wasted —that if in the professional estimation of NIH officials money provided would not buy progress and scientific competence, they would not spend it. Hence the committees could confidently appropriate generously for NIH because of the managerial controls, based on scientific integrity, imposed by Dr. Shannon.[9]

The situation obtaining in the late sixties, however, even if it followed an old, occasionally recurring dollar pattern, was not a matter of stringent use of NIH controls, or of a budgetary disagreement based on philosophical differences among the agency, the Congress, and the President about whether too much was being spent too fast. It was, rather, that the war had produced such a shortage of dollars that the most willing presidential spender in modern history was forced to hold back on spending for some of the programs he most believed in.

In the new and difficult context, the intensified, increasingly bitter fight among parties of the old medical research coalition, reflecting increasing certainty on the part of each that it was right about ends and means, further retarded the cause. Once the fight was recognized, of course, some tried to cast all new developments in terms of that struggle. And trying to prove the very old case that Congress "force fed NIH" became a lively sport among Washington-based reporters. But if exaggerations of purposes and cross-purposes occurred, it was the fault of the coalition members, not the press.

An instance of congressional initiative in 1967 became a front-page story in the *Washington Post* of September 3:

> The National Institutes of Health, one of few agencies on
> which Capitol Hill regularly showers more money than it
> requests, may get $4 million it did not seek this year for a
> heart drug study it did not recommend . . .
>
> Senator Lister Hill (D., Ala.) was so impressed by testi-
> monials on the new drugs prospects that he dropped the $4
> million into the NIH money bill at the last minute without
> bothering to get the views of the agency that would spend
> it—NIH's National Heart Institute.

The first part of the story, for those who had followed the history of the congressional role in the development of the national
medical research enterprise, was not new. The last part was. By
the accounts of both Hill and Shannon, as well as of committee
clerks, agency staff, and inside lobbyists, rarely if ever had a
new program or research direction been foisted upon the
agency without clear advance notice and mutual discussion,
even if the agency was sometimes reluctant.

The matter at issue, according to the *Post* story, was the possibility of a new study of a drug called Atromid-S, which had already been shown to lower the level of cholesterol and other
fatty substances in the bloodstream. During the course of that
portion of the Senate subcommittee's hearings when citizen witnesses appeared, Dr. Jessie Marmorston (clinical professor of
medicine at the University of California, whose work had attracted Mrs. Lasker's attention and support) and two of her colleagues described a possible study of whether the drug tended
to prevent heart attacks. Dr. DeBakey seemed to think this a
good idea. Senator Hill, the only Senator present at that moment, didn't remember that Atromid-S was one of five drugs being tested in a similar study already under way under the Heart
Institute's auspices, and he directed that $4 million be added to
the Institute's appropriation to conduct such a study as that described.[10]

The full committee and the Senate itself went along, as usual, with the appropriations proposed by the Senator from Alabama. But the House of Representatives balked; it rejected the first conference report the House managers of the Labor-HEW appropriations bill brought back from their meeting with their Senate counterparts. Indeed, the House instructed its conferees not to come back with a report containing any more money for NIH than what the House had agreed to in the first place. (And that was $3 million less than the Bureau of the Budget had approved.) The House prevailed, and a pattern which had been in effect for almost 20 years was broken. One of the meanings of the change was that there would be no special, "unrequested" study of Atromid-S.

In the 20 fiscal years from 1948 to 1968, the House of Representatives on 16 occasions voted more money for the National Institutes of Health than the President had asked for. Three times during that period—twice in the years of the Korean War and again for 1968—the House reduced the budget request for NIH, and once (for 1963) it accepted the budget exactly as presented by the executive. John Fogarty presided over one budget cut (but only of $1 million in 1950) and helped his friend Jack Kennedy keep the budget down for 1963, following the President's special request to him. Every year save one during the same period, the Senate not only increased the President's budget for medical research, but went beyond whatever increases the House had included. In 20 years, only four times— 1951, 1952, 1964, and 1968—did Congress ultimately fail to provide more for NIH than what the President, through the Bureau of the Budget, thought was adequate. For those four years, the reductions Congress made were from $1 million to $6 million.

For the other 16 years, the pattern was that the House would raise the figure by several million dollars ($50 or $60 million in a "good year") and the Senate by many millions more (almost $200 million in 1962); then the conferees would work out a figure somewhere in between. Some House members complained that the final figure was usually closer to the high Senate figure than to that approved by the House. That was not actually the case; sometimes the amount agreed upon by the conferees was closer to the Senate preference (1954, 1957, 1965) and sometimes to the House figure (1963, 1964). Most of the time the difference was split right down the middle. In that way, without any spoken agreement between them, Fogarty and Hill in a kind of de facto collusion lifted medical research appropriations to new, unexpected heights.

In the year that Senator Hill tried to push the Atromid-S special study, he found a changed situation in the House. His longtime, stalwart if formally unacknowledged ally John Fogarty was dead. Fogarty's successor, Daniel J. Flood (D., Pa.), brought to his new position the advantages of having had a personal, recurring brush with the enemy—cancer—and a dramatic presence shaped by earlier performances on the legitimate stage. In the first years of his new chairmanship, he did not have the grasp of facts or the parliamentary skills, the tenacity in debate, or the personal support of the Irish brigade that Fogarty had developed. Congressman Laird offered what help he could, although he was not insistent that the House committee raise the budget figures. The *Washington Post* story about the Hill-Marmorston-Lasker-DeBakey attempt at another end run to start the Atromid-S study did not help matters.

In addition to war-produced budget strains, the absence of the old pro John Fogarty, and one more example of the Senate's incorrigible zeal, the Cause received another blow. In November 1967, before the House-Senate conference report on NIH appropriations for fiscal 1968 had been finally resolved, the Fountain Committee fired another salvo at NIH management.[11] The combination of events made it virtually impossible for Dan Flood to keep up the momentum, the traditional pattern.

Just a few months after President Johnson appraised the NIH as "a billion-dollar success story" (thus removed himself from direct aim of the barbs and arrows of outraged scientists whose research grant fortunes were threatened) the Fountain Committee brought its most serious charges of the decade against the medical research agency. It charged the agency with "weak central management," with concentrating grants in a small group of institutions and by doing so widening the gap in the biosciences between "rich" and "poor" schools, with "inept handling" of reimbursements to grantees of indirect costs, and with general "laxity" in the administration of grants to institutions of higher education. But it reserved its most serious and elaborate attack, in the 113-page catalogue of deficiencies against the Institutes and the Public Health Service, on just that aspect of the agency's modus operandi and values that Dr. Shannon was proudest of and bragged most about: the quality of the scientists and research projects supported.[12]

In the Committee's judgment, NIH was spending far too great sums of money to support too many research projects, a large proportion of which were "lower than good quality." [13] (Whether this related to NIH's attempts, and President Johnson's desire, to support research at a wider variety and geographical placement of institutions and get away from an elitist pattern of geographic concentration—which the Committee also criticized—is not something the Committee bothered to explore or comment on.) Specifically, the Fountain Committee found very unhealthy and ill-advised NIH's commitment to the Sloan-Kettering Cancer Institute of a "block grant" for support of its scientists' work, entailing a "moral commitment" to the Institute to continue the support for a five-year period. The move on the agency's part was designed to meet the increasing demand—born of the frustration of a fragmented, halting process that forestalled a coordinated, sustained attack on the basic causes of disease and exploration of the basic elements of science—for a more sustained fiscal commitment. And such a move was related to the desires of members of Congress like Senator Margaret Smith for long-range planning, as well as to the urgings of grant recipients. Still, such a commitment, despite being only "moral," made government accountants and HEW lawyers nervous, for the law precludes the obligation of public funds before they are actually appropriated by the people's elected representatives in Congress. Aside from that issue, the Fountain Committee zeroed in on the quality of the work of Sloan-Kettering scientists, finding that quality, according to NIH's own evaluations of the recent past, by no means universally high. During a two-and-a-half year period on which Fountain Committee investigators focused, 20 out of 34 applications submitted individually by Sloan-Kettering scientists were rejected—a less than breathtaking batting average. The Committee reported that Sloan-Kettering had supported some research projects which NIH, despite its usual posture of extraordinary generosity, had turned down because its advisers thought they lacked scientific merit.[14]

In short, concentrating on Shannon's early and continuing insistence that the only critically important aspect of grant-giving was in picking the right man to do the right research, and his repeated claim that NIH's record on that score was unimpeachable whatever other kinds of management weaknesses might exist, Fountain believed he had finally separated theory from fact. He hoped he had punctured the bloated mystique about the inherent integrity of science and the essential triviality of good management practices.

Even in the judgment of friends of NIH, this was the strongest case the Fountain Committee had made against the research agency.[15] Fountain wanted to make sure its broader implications were not lost on his colleagues. He still believed that a central problem was that Congress had been "overzealous in appropriating money for health research," and that such pressure as that created was responsible for the agency's inability to keep up with the problems of basic management.[16] And he suggested that if the President really wanted to save money and reduce unnecessary federal expenditures, he should turn his attention to waste in health research funds.

This time, there were two signal differences in the way NIH

responded to its congressional critic. First, it did not undertake to mount its defense alone, but rather allowed the parent Department to coordinate the effort to overcome the potentially damaging effects of Fountain's charges. Secretary John Gardner transmitted the analysis and comment to the Committee. Second, while staunch defense was made of the agency on many issues raised by the Committee, and specific rebuttal offered on some points, the tone of the response was diplomatic and unemotional. Secretary Gardner said that the Department had "no disagreement in substance" with 14 out of 17 of the Committee's recommendations. Nonetheless, reported the correspondent for *Science*, "a closer reading of the report itself reveals that NIH stands firmly behind the actions that brought about Fountain's most stinging accusations" (March 1, 1968, p. 959).

Dr. Shannon's response, commented Philip Abelson, editor of *Science*, was "dignified and thoughtful." [17] There was, this time, nothing in the reply that could be considered by Congress as arrogant or condescending. The problem now was that many people had already chosen sides, had divided into what Abelson a year and a half later plainly labeled "advocates and opponents of medical research." [18] With the advocates' bloc shrinking and divided, and the swing group in Congress increasingly small, increasingly important, and increasingly persuadable by arguments of the opponents, it is no wonder that the House cut NIH appropriations by $40 million the year after the Fountain Committee report of October 1967. The Johnson Administration had not indicated any loss of faith; in fact both HEW and the Bureau of the Budget made smaller cuts in the estimates of fiscal need suggested by the Institutes than in any recent year. Nor had Lister Hill lost confidence or spunk. Once more, and for the last time, he led the Senate in raising the proposed appropriations for the National Institutes of Health, in the summer of 1968, by more than $50 million over the House-approved figure and $10 million over the Budget Bureau allowance. The final appropriation for fiscal 1969, however, was $1.1 billion. In the wake of John Fogarty's death and L. H. Fountain's onslaught, Congress cut the NIH budget by almost $20 million—the largest cut the agency had sustained in its history, and the first time Congress had indicated genuine skepticism about medical research.[19]

1968 marked the end of a remarkable era in government, in science, and in social and political history. For medical research the passing of that year was like passing into a condition of political orphanage. Lister Hill, like Lyndon Johnson, chose not to run for re-election. Politics were becoming increasingly difficult for moderates in Alabama; that, plus Mrs. Hill's uncertain health, moved the Senator to his decision. Besides, he thought 45 years' service in Congress was enough.

James Shannon, who had guided NIH through 13 years of political and scientific *bouleversement* to the plateau of its greatest importance, also retired that year. Although his successor, Dr. Robert Q. Marston, had the advantage of a strong, thoughtful, and experienced NIH administrator—Dr. John F. Sherman —as his general Deputy Director, and Dr. Shannon's longtime collaborator—Dr. Robert W. Berliner—as Deputy Director for Science, the new Director himself did not possess the aura of strength, independence, and purposefulness which his predecessor had always radiated.

President Johnson's replacement by Richard Nixon meant the substitution of a known friend of health, if a skeptical supporter of basic biomedical research, by a largely unknown factor. President Nixon's unknown attitude toward the biomedical science enterprise was all the more worrisome for believers in the Cause because of his known proclivity for balanced budgets. His appointment of Congressman Laird as Secretary of Defense was further cause for concern, for Laird had become a staunch friend of the enterprise.

Mary Lasker and Florence Mahoney, volunteered one commentator, were "no longer young women." [20] If true, no sign of age was reflected in their continuing extraordinary activities in the crusade to improve the health of the people of the planet Earth, especially America. Mrs. Lasker renewed her efforts to secure enactment of a comprehensive national health insurance plan. And Mrs. Mahoney stepped up her at-home tutorials on the latest biomedical knowledge and how to take advantage of it, on plausible if not yet popular possibilities in biomedical engineering, and on the probable political good fortune of those—specifically, the new members of her "seminars" who were mainly new members of Congress—who espoused and promoted health programs. The two crusaders were hampered, of course, by the loss of allies in Congress and frustrated by lack of friends in the White House. But the principal personal disadvantage the new Administration caused them was that, when their terms expired on Institute Advisory Councils in 1970, neither was reappointed. For Mrs. Lasker, it was the first time in 18 years that she had not been able to sit among the councils of scientists and physicians, to learn from them the latest bioscience lessons while instructing them in the fundamental purposes of the enterprise and exploring with them the best means of achieving them. Some thought the medical research lobby was through.

Whether events and causes make men, or instead men move and make the forces of history, is an ancient, recurrent issue. Perhaps construction of the greatest medical research empire in the world is a significant enough contribution to man's collective advance that the question can be examined again, without exaggeration and with prospects for an answer, in that delimited context.

No clear answers quickly emerge. Indeed, it is almost as though there are two separate histories of the "billion-dollar-plus success story" represented by the rise of the National Institutes of Health at the center of the empire. One history is recorded in sweeping terms of national interests developing out of national experience. It highlights, first, a remarkable but coincidental convergence of dramatic world and national events, of war and the medical science successes and new governmental arrangements it produced; of unleashed scientific talent attracted by newly emergent medical possibilities, interspersed with critical basic knowledge gaps; of a natural turning toward problems within the nation, including those within human beings—then of fears invigorated by continuing international rivalries; and of the willingness of citizens and their elected spokesmen to continue to spend great sums of money for important common causes based on common fears. This history suggests that there were forces, needs, desires, and challenges at work that inexorably combined to produce great new national enterprises, regardless of which personalities rode the crest of the building wave.

The other history is a highly personalized one. It emphasizes the prescience and persistence of Mary Lasker, the political power and skill and the compassion of Lister Hill and John Fogarty, and the extraordinary and felicitous combination of scientific integrity and organizational leadership of James Shannon. Other persons and groups provided crucial assists at various critical junctures. But without these particular individuals, this version implies, the outcome of this small segment of history would be enormously different.

In weighing the importance of single persons on the course of a national policy, and in that sense on the course of history, perhaps it is enough to know that some are perceived as giants. In the politics of medical research Hill, Fogarty, Lasker, Mahoney, Shannon, and several others certainly are.

In the eyes of his colleagues in the House of Representative, John Fogarty was not just a fellow trying hard to keep abreast of an exuberant throng. He was a leader, and a formidable opponent. He was virtually the only subcommittee chairman of the House Appropriations Committee, colleagues recall, who regularly stood up against a tough chairman and tough rules about spending, and regularly won. Part of the reason, they admit, was that Fogarty was onto a good thing. But much more important, he "did his homework" by marshaling all the evidence and by lining up some support from his colleagues in advance. It was obvious that Fogarty enjoyed the special stature the Cause gave him, and sought to use it to political advantage back home; but that would not have persuaded colleagues to accept his leadership. What did, in personal terms, was that in addition to his impressive analysis of all relevant facts, he *believed*. Heavy discount must always be made in assessing the meaning of public compliments passed around among congressional colleagues; but the venerable Sam Rayburn's estimation of John Fogarty's successful floor fight to increase funds for medical research in 1954 as "one of the most powerful and convincing speeches and arguments that I have listened to since I have become a member of this House" was beyond the usual laurel-tossing. For, as Rayburn remarked, "I am not given to complimenting people on this floor, as everybody who has served with me knows." [21] Nor was there any discernible political motivation for the compliment offered by Representative Charles A. Wolverton (R., N.J.), sometime chairman of the House Interstate and Foreign Commerce Committee, about Fogarty in 1957: "The gentleman from Rhode Island leaves no doubt that he is the best informed man in Congress on all details affecting our national health program." [22] Well informed, thought Congressman George Mahon (D., Texas), but indiscriminately generous when it comes to medical research. Mahon, chairman of the full House Appropriations Committee, had as much trouble keeping subcommittee chairman Fogarty "in line" as did his predecessor, Clarence Cannon. "The trouble with John," remarked Mr. Mahon, "was that he wanted to give NIH *everything but* the Capitol dome." [23]

Lister Hill, said his unhappy colleague Senator Paul Douglas (D., Ill.), who was having a hard time getting what he wanted out of a parliamentary situation while the senior Senator from Alabama was doing quite well, "is so persuasive, so charming, so quietly indispensable, and so personally self-effacing, that

we want to give him everything that it is possible to give him."
There were of course various reasons, both general and particular, why the Senate always supported medical research in a big
way, but as far as Senator Douglas was concerned, "the National Institutes of Health owe their extremely flowering condition to the Senator from Alabama . . . He touches the rock of
public credit and abundant streams gush forth so that the National Institutes of Health have money running out of their ears,
money they do not always know what to do with." [24]

Some doctor-scientists are said to be impressed with the fact
that Mrs. Lasker knows more about biomedicine than many of
their colleagues. Mainly however, the genius she is most credited with is that which Dr. DeBakey specified: "She has a quick
mind, an ability to focus on the central issues and to sense what
combination of talents must be brought together to solve a
problem." [25] A federal official is credited with saying that
throughout the two decades of effort to build the medical research enterprise, including periods of controversy, Mary Lasker "has been almost always right." [26] The implication, of course,
is that some of her critics and opponents within government
have often been wrong. According to Senator Hill, Mrs. Lasker's
unique contribution is that "she has sounded the alarm that
made it possible for us to get the support to do the things we
have done." [27]

Most of James Shannon's scientific colleagues whose associations with the national medical research story relate to their being on the receiving end or in the supervisory middle consider
Shannon the most important single figure in the entire enterprise. It was he, after all, who stood in the center of it and directed with firm command what they perceive to be the most
difficult aspect of any national policy: producing the desired
results.

It is not necessarily informing of the answer to the main question, but it is a not uninteresting fact, that the unquestionably
important individuals who initiated and shaped national medi-

cal research policy from the immediate postwar years to 1970 *believe* that they were responsible for bringing us much closer to a Golden Age of Medicine than we could otherwise possibly be. Theirs is not a perspective inclining toward the theory of natural evolution of national endeavors. They are convinced that progress is only made when purposeful and determined persons are relentlessly guiding it. Mrs. Lasker's credo is based on the observation of Maurice Maeterlinck: "At every crossing on the road that leads to the future, each progressive spirit is opposed by a thousand men appointed to guard the past." [28]

There is, as well, evidence that each group leader involved in the great alliance that built the medical research empire believes his to have been the most crucial role. Lister Hill's acknowledgment that Mrs. Lasker, Mrs. Mahoney, and their friends "sounded the alarm" is an introductory phrase the main predicate of which is, "we [in Congress] did the job." Mrs. Lasker agrees on the important role of Hill and Fogarty, indeed emphasizes it in conversation. But what is also clear is that her "outside lobbyists" believe that, along with her, they have been the principal catalyst and driving force behind the alliance.

At one point in his earlier career at NIH, Dr. Shannon would have admitted that the power and purpose lay with the two congressional committees (and two members of Congress specifically) and the citizens lobby (and Mrs. Lasker specifically).[29] Looking back on the enterprise he has left, Dr. Shannon now seems inclined to give little credit to the Lasker-Mahoney group. When asked about support he sometimes needed and elicited from the outside, he thinks principally of figures in science whose names are unconnected with the prominent medical research activists. Moreover, he seems to have withdrawn a previously stated view that the citizens groups were a key factor in moving the effort forward; in considering the matter retrospectively, he emphasizes their misguided meddling in the internal operations of the research agency, their unfortunate and damaging insistence on trying to move too fast on a range of delicate matters, from development of artificial hearts to field trials for certain drugs.

Shannon's present view is that Congress was both understanding and helpful in a supportive way, which was fortunate given the executive branch's lack of interest. But Congress was not in a dominant position: Shannon never simply carried out the wishes of the policy makers in Congress, nor did the Hill and Fogarty committees limit his freedom in management in any significant degree. It is Marion Folsom and John Gardner whom Shannon thinks of first as being among the more important contributors to national medical research policy over the last two decades (after all, each of them backed him in difficult situations). Of course, some of the institute directors were terribly conservative; and there were some in the science community who lacked ability to adjust to the new ways and pace of research and who had to be either goosed along or dropped by the wayside.[30] In summary, it was the NIH directorate that guided and supervised the construction, devising its own "master plan" as it went along, absorbing and utilizing occasional boosts and deflecting occasional barbs from outside, and finally putting in place the system which would deliver the policy results it had principally posited. In a word, it was Shannon who did it.

In Mrs. Lasker's judgment, Dr. Shannon's inherent conservatism and his ego, which caused him to be increasingly unreceptive to ideas of others, are factors in what she believes is a recent period of disappointing progress. She does not claim to have possessed over-riding power; she confesses, sadly, that in those several struggles in which she represented one point of view and Shannon the opposite—struggles over pace and direction, she insists, not over control of internal management—she almost always lost.[31] She had immediate access to the President as well as to the key members of Congress. Surgeons General, to whom Dr. Shannon officially reported, who were sometimes appointed at the suggestion of Mary Lasker or some of her friends and who sometimes resigned because they couldn't get to see the

Secretary of HEW or the President while she always could, thought she had too easy access and too much influence. But she couldn't necessarily translate that access and influence into victories over particular issues. Yet if she did not come out on top in a power struggle, she considers herself right on the principles. She would claim no particular brilliance, and would deny she had power, but she would not disagree with the assessment that "she has been an indispensable mobilizer of public and congressional will." [32] Indeed, worrying over the relative paucity of practical health results after 15 years of heavy federal investment in medical research, Mrs. Lasker concludes that the reason must be that "I did something wrong—or didn't do enough of the right things." [33] Thus, graciously accepting personal responsibility for its shortcomings, she firmly places herself, in retrospect, in a central position in the national medical research enterprise.

In Senator Hill's judgment, many people were "very helpful." Mrs. Lasker, Mrs. Mahoney, Mike Gorman, Margaret Chase Smith, Norris Cotton, John Pastore, Michael DeBakey, Sidney Farber, several NIH scientists and officials, and a number of others must be credited, in Hill's view, with contributing importantly to the development of an advanced state of medical research in America today. John Fogarty was "*very, very* helpful." Very, very helpful, Hill says, but apparently he did not think Fogarty was crucial. He does not say whether anyone was, but lets it rest thus: "A lot of people helped me." [34]

John Fogarty used lay and physician witnesses as "window dressing"; he conferred with Dr. Shannon frequently; he lined up support from House colleagues on votes; he acknowledged the signal importance of Melvin Laird; and he expected Senator Hill, "a nice fellow," [35] to increase the appropriation for medical research over whatever he proposed. Everybody knew it was tougher to get increases in the House than in the Senate; Fogarty's contribution, for that reason, was greater than Hill's, say many of Fogarty's friends and some seemingly neutral analysts.

Meanwhile, Fogarty took his cues from the institute directors' "professional judgments," decided what research need to emphasize in a given year, then proceeded to orchestrate the other elements around his chosen theme.

In truth, each of the powerful personalities (and each of the three baronies that made up the triune force) played crucial roles. Each was the product of all his days. Together they established policy, wrote history. Different circumstances might have replaced them with other individuals; but that they are responsible for launching and accelerating an important national effort is as clear as that their task was made easier by a conducive environment.

What also became clearer as the dust from the 1968–69 presidential transition settled down was that the medical research enterprise was still largely intact, if nonetheless in trouble. The Nixon Administration seemed certain to be more conservative fiscally than its predecessor; its proposed budgets for NIH for fiscal 1970 (the first budget prepared by the Nixon Administration) was $35 million below the previous year's appropriation, and that for fiscal 1971 $20 million below what Congress had approved a year earlier. This Administration has followed one lead opened by Johnson: increasing the effort, and the money, for finding "breakthroughs" while indicating less than enchantment with basic research.

But if the Nixon Administration is not altogether enthusiastic about the total medical research enterprise, it will not be the first one to assume that posture. Meanwhile, there are some signs that congressional interest, and congressional bipartisanship, is reviving after a bad year for the Cause following the last Fountain Committee attack and the departure of Fogarty and Hill.

Dan Flood flexed his muscles slightly in the House in 1970, producing and securing acceptance of a budget for NIH $2 million over the President's request. Further, the bipartisan coalition on the House committee bubbled with potential revival.

Representative Bob Michel (R., Ill.)—who once said on the floor of the House (to the chagrin of chairman Fogarty, who had just claimed that his committee always produced unanimous reports) that he was in disagreement with appropriations figures recommended by the committee,[36] and on another occasion said he had usually voted against the Labor-HEW appropriations bill because he thought it was too big[37]—became a notable ally. It was Michel who explained to the House what cystic fibrosis was, and Michel who urged the House to support the chairman and the committee in approving the appropriation that went above the President's budget.[38]

On the Senate side, Warren (Maggie) Magnuson (D., Wash.) took over the chairmanship vacated by Senator Hill. A good sign—and if that was not sufficiently clear, Maggie made it clearer when the first witnesses came to discuss the appropriations for NIH for 1970. He reminded them that he had been one of the pioneers in developing the federal involvement in health as (he said) the original sponsor of the Cancer Bill back in 1937.[39] (Senator Hill had never failed to acknowledge Magnuson's early involvement in the Cause: "He swam out and found that the water was fine, and ever since then some of the rest of us have been going in." [40]) In the first year of his new job, with the cooperation of Senator Cotton, Magnuson added $112 million to the President's proposal for NIH and $100 million more than the House had secured under the new team of Flood and Michel. The final figure appropriated was $56 million more than the executive had requested.

Moreover, a new constituency began to emerge, which gave evidence that it would fight cuts in medical research budgets and possibly fight for increases. It was principally comprised of the university-science community—the group that had been the longtime, long-silent beneficiary of governmental largesse in research funds. In a rare call to arms, *Science* outlined the situation as regards friends (Senator Magnuson, Senator Cotton, possibly Secretary of Health, Education and Welfare, Robert

Finch), and foes (possibly the whole House committee and definitely the Bureau of the Budget).[41] Not only had the Bureau "worked over" the NIH budget for 1970, said *Science*, cutting it by $100 million, but it might well inflict further cuts by putting a ceiling on research expenditures regardless of what Congress appropriated. The editorial concluded: "If scientists wish to comment on support of medical research, they should address their letters of praise to Senator Magnuson and their complaints to President Nixon."

Such communications as the Congress received no doubt encouraged its addition of another $56 million for NIH that year. The following year, for fiscal 1971, Congress increased the President's budget by almost $100 million, giving the agency a nine-percent increase in research funds over the previous year; and for 1972, the House and Senate health appropriations subcommittees added over $140 million to the President's request. A sizable portion of that increase was for research on aging, an area which Senator Magnuson had been convinced (by his longtime friend Florence Mahoney) was very important and had been theretofore neglected.

The medical research lobby might have lost some of its force; the old coalition which comprised that lobby, the congressional committees, and the NIH was no longer as visible or as viable as in earlier days. But there were signs that new forces were gathering to carry on. The national medical research enterprise, it seemed, regardless of whose initiatives and nurturing had gotten it launched and moving, had developed a life and momentum of its own.

XI An Assessment of Policy Results

What constitutes national policy is a debatable and much-debated issue. National policy is usually recognized as such when it is synoptically developed and/or presidentially enunciated. Thus there was no question, after President John F. Kennedy's declaration in 1961 that we would attempt to land a man on the moon before the end of the decade, what our space policy would be for that period. On the other hand, even presidentially stated intentions, if no consistent effort is made to implement them, may not be tantamount to governmental policy. Further, even when national goals are stated and accepted, and machinery is set up to achieve them, functional policy with a constant lifeline may not result.

Sometimes specific policies fail, but those who might feel incriminated by accepting the verdict of failure voice the view that "we never really had a policy." Avowed critics of particular national policies also sometimes refuse to admit that policy makers have made policy. Their charge that no policy exists suggests that confusion does; and that is considered to be as damning an indictment as the assessment that there is a policy but that it is wrong.

In the case of the national medical research enterprise over the last 20 years, critics of various aspects and with varying motives have often commented that there is no government policy. What is apparently meant by that charge is that there has been no centrally issued, widely promulgated summary statement of what nonetheless has developed into an unmistakable governmental commitment. The charge may also reflect some divergence of view about what the main thrusts of the policy were and should be. Some—notably those in the executive branch of government—have simply been bothered about calling anything a policy that emanates largely from legislative concerns and actions.

If we accept policy making as "essentially an ordering of priorities," [1] we can accept the possibility that policy may either be made according to a logical, synoptic process necessitating explicit agreement and goals, or that policy can evolve out of a series of marginal moves and uncoordinated decisions, permitted by vague agreement on broad goals but not necessitating specific accords or ordered sequences of actions. Policy, that is, can evolve de facto out of an aggregate of decisions and commitments only indirectly related to one another.

National medical research policy has not been characterized, in the past quarter century, by a strictly logical, purely synoptic decision-making process. But it has been relatively coherent, relatively consistent, and relatively plain. The first efforts to formulate it, the boldest plans for it, the strongest sustaining moves, and the clearest statement of its goals and components were provided by Congress. The Senate Appropriations Subcommittee, chaired by Senator Edward Thye (R., Minn.), stated in 1950 what it called "policy guides":

> Upon consideration . . . of the general development of medical research in this country, the committee reaffirms what it believes to be the general policy guides upon which decisions on Federal appropriations should rest. These are 1) adequate support for promising scientific investigations relating to knowledge of disease which cannot be aided from other sources, and 2) expansion of the national pool of trained medical scientists to permit an expanded medical research effort in the future.[2]

Under Senator Hill's chairmanship, the committee elaborated the nature and purposes of the policy in its 1960 report to the Senate:

In essence, though it has not been so stated, there has come into being a national policy that calls for a sustained and expanded research attack against disease. Under that policy the Federal Government has assumed a share of the total responsibility for a strong medical research effort, as reflected primarily in increased appropriations for the activities of the National Institutes of Health.

. . . Congressional action taken in connection with these appropriations is the most important decision affecting medical research in the Nation and has a profound though indirect effect on the education processes in our schools that train our physicians, dentists and other health professionals. Moreover, because of the work supported, the scientists trained, and the institutional stability engendered by a consistent pattern of congressional support, the action of Congress on these appropriations determines in no small measure the rate of acquisition of new knowledge which will lead to a more precise understanding of the nature of the many fatal or disabling diseases which afflict our people, thus hastening the day when these may be prevented, cured, or ameliorated.[3]

In short, the ultimate goal was to control and if possible "conquer" disease, thereby improving the people's health. To attain that goal, an intermediary goal was understood: the biomedical research enterprise must be built up, and institutions and individual researchers supported. That, in turn, would require great amounts of money, and Congress thought the government should be willing to spend it.

What have been the results of that policy? Has it succeeded, or failed, or merely muddled along?

Judging the success or failure of national policies is a difficult proposition. As in questioning whether there is a policy to begin with, some will define success so as to prove that it has or has not been achieved, according to their agreement or disagreement with the policy in the first place. Beyond that, except where policy goals are narrowly discrete, unchanging, and "one-time," standards of measurement may necessarily be largely suggestive. (When Armstrong, Aldrin, and Collins reached and returned from the moon, there was no question that a specific goal had been attained.) In most policy areas, even when broad purposes remain constant, component targets may shift, expand, or contract according to new needs and new knowledge constantly emerging. Just as those who participate in the development of a national policy can only be described, especially in a democracy, as "proximate policy makers" because each is one of many—so ordinarily should we only expect that a given policy will proximately attain posited goals.

The National Biomedical Science Network

It seems clear that the conscious, consistent, heavy support of biomedical research by the federal government over the past two decades has produced one of the goals desired by the policy makers. Straddling the broad areas of health and science, of research sponsorship and support for other higher education functions, national medical research policy has resulted in the construction of a biomedical research system of great size and enormous importance. The enterprise of which NIH is the central source was supporting, at its peak in 1967–68, more than 67,000 senior research investigators; it sustains academic science programs and research projects in more than 2,000 universities and medical schools, and helps provide advanced science training in basic science and various clinical specialties for more than 35,-000 individuals.

The science establishment, including the NIH directorate over the years, particularly wished to create such a system. They would have preferred another means of determining proper funding levels, to insure that the flow of funds be steady, not too fast, and never retrogressive. The science directorate believed that, ideally, *they* should decide how much money was needed and how many researchers should be engaged in which pursuits. In an ideal world, the first preference of the science establishment, including the NIH directorate, would have been to let the biomedical science managers direct the enterprise in an unfettered way—unfettered, that is, by the pressures that always affect the allocation of resources in a democracy.

Still, Dr. Shannon indicated he did not feel threatened by the political context in which he had to operate in the early 1960's. At that point, the context was generally supportive of his aims and, in any case, ultimately permitted him and his in-house and outside advisers to pursue goals they thought were of paramount importance. Asked in 1961 whether he thought NIH should be given the status of an independent agency, Shannon replied:

> I feel we are in a protected position where, by and large, I and my immediate staff can address ourselves to the needs of the nation as encompassed in our programs, to the professional character of our programs, to the interplay between our programs and the university world, without worrying about the political overlay that becomes an essential part of our total operation as soon as it is placed in a more publicly sensitive position.
>
> I am using politics in the best sense of the word, in the sense that, as the Army must be governed by civilians, so science must be governed in the final analysis by non-scientists. When we compete for dollars within the Federal budget, the decision as to how much comes to us, and as to how much goes elsewhere, is in a broad sense a political decision.[4]

At that particular point in time, Shannon summed up his position thus: "So I have certain vested interests, of a personal nature, in retaining the status quo."

Subsequent pressures from Congress and the medical re-

search lobby altered his attitude somewhat. In the very real political world, Dr. Shannon did not expect to be totally free of accountability. He simply would have preferred an arrangement
whereby executive reviewers would allow him to determine the
proper scientific course and the proper pace of pursuing it, then
back him all the way as the political process ensued.

The science establishment believed that the only way to approach the ultimate policy goal—"the improvement of virtually
all aspects of the Nation's health"—was simply by "the stimulation and support of a very broad range of health-related or biomedical research." [5] That that mission has been carried out is
obvious, and that the system created for carrying it out is a permanent fixture on the national policy landscape is only slightly
less obvious. The broad scientific work goes on within the elaborate and extensive governmental support system, and within
the government laboratories.

The system sometimes seems a little shaky, but the work performed within it has received near-universal acclaim. Every
study of the National Institutes of Health and the research it
supports—from the friendly Jones Commitee Report to the apparently neutral studies of the Woolridge Committee and the
American Medical Association's Whittaker Commission to the
critical Fountain Committee—has concluded that, whatever
faults there may be with present operational aspects or whatever needs there may be for the future, the scientific quality of
work performed under NIH auspices has been high.

The Woolridge Committee documented its finding that "the
large majority of the intramural and extramural research supported by NIH is of high quality." Specifically, it reported that
its "panel teams" had looked at 240 extramural research grants,
expressing reservations about only nine and adjudging seven
"unworthy of support." That, said the Committee, was an im-
pressively low ratio of ill-advised projects. Moreover, the group
stated, frequently "NIH-supported work was found to set the
national or international standard of excellence in its field." Fur-

ther, the Committee found that, as federal funds were increasing between 1955 and 1965, so the average quality of work supported was attaining higher levels.[6]

Joseph D. Cooper, commenting on the Woolridge Report, noted that many of those who participate in the "panel team" assessments are themselves sometime NIH grantees.[7] But Cooper, who was a consultant to the Whittaker Commission of the AMA and who had an important hand in writing the Whittaker Report, concedes that the NIH should be given credit for doing "a tremendous job."[8] Officially, the AMA commission summarized one of its conclusions thus: "We concur in the general belief that the current level of adequacy and excellence of our biomedical research resources has never before been equalled, although it is probable that the abundant Federal funds for research have inescapably supported a measure of mediocrity as well as the nation's best scientific talent."[9]

There is other evidence that the goal of a surpassingly good medical science-research establishment has been achieved. In the past 20 years the already developing trend of medical science looking to the United States rather than to Europe has become an accepted fact: today the United States is the acknowledged leader in science, including the biomedical sciences, in the West and many would say in the world. The rate of Nobel Prize winners in physiology and medicine has changed dramatically in favor of the United States in recent years. The research of 41 Americans winning the Nobel Prize in those two areas in the last 25 years has been supported by the National Institutes of Health; two recent Nobel laureates—Marshall Nirenberg in 1968 and Julius Axelrod in 1970—have performed their research in the intramural program of NIH.

By far the largest aggregate activity of the National Institutes of Health is that occurring outside the agency, under grants and contracts which support research and related activities by individual scientists and institutions. But the intramural program is crucially important to the enterprise. Carrying on the tradition of the Hygienic Laboratory, NIH has eight intramural divisions which today house the world's largest and most diversified concentration of biomedical investigators.

Tensions have occasionally arisen between those who favored strengthening, and increasing the size, of the research effort within the NIH and those who wanted to keep it small—because they thought it merely extended the conservative microbiologist syndrome of earlier years, or because they thought the best way to secure popular support for biomedical science was to spread financial support around. Generally speaking, the desire to strengthen the intramural effort has been largely an intra-agency sentiment and the desire to keep that effort small while expanding the extramural effort a position favored by constituencies outside the agency, for once including actively and together both the medical research lobby and the university scientists and science administrators. In that situation, for example, restrictions have been placed on the eligibility of intramural scientists to compete for extramural awards for research and training support; and the expert panels providing advice on various aspects of the extramural programs have, by design, included relatively few in-house experts at any given time.

Most observers would agree that combination of internal and external research and clinical activities of the NIH is a healthy one, and that both features of the NIH system have contributed to the strong national biomedical research system that exists today. The intramural pool of scientists has been a primary source of program leadership for the agency; and large numbers of scientists now located at various institutions around the country, as well as many academic officers of graduate and health professional schools, have spent portions of their careers as members of the NIH staff.

The Conquest of Disease

How close national medical research policy has brought us to the central goal of conquering disease is a more difficult matter to judge then whether a first-rate biomedical science system has been created. Yet no one has been known to dispute the broad statement of Dr. John A. D. Cooper, president of the Association of American Medical Colleges, that knowledge accumulated over a twenty-year period has "revolutionized the range of diagnostic, therapeutic and preventive capabilities of medicine," and has made it possible for physicians to offer more favorable prognoses to patients suffering from many diseases.[10] The Jones Committee of 1960 asserted that "the expanding program of medical research has made tremendous contributions to medical practice . . . and has been a prime factor in raising the standard of medical care to the highest level ever achieved." [11]

Some analysts are dubious that recent health gains have stemmed from only slightly less recent medical research expenditures. "The truth of the matter," said the Whittaker Commission, is that "striking increases in life expectancy and changes in the profile of disease . . . stem from earlier periods preceding the current effort." Yet the Commission concluded: "There is hardly an aspect of medical practice which has not been enriched in some way as a result of advancement in biomedical science." [12] Dr. Walsh McDermott of Cornell reminds us that public health measures have contributed to health improvement as significantly as medical research measures have.[13] And Elizabeth Drew suggests that "a great many more deaths might be prevented, or diseases cured if smoking were reduced, if automobiles were safer, if the air were cleaner, than through post-facto disease-oriented research and services." [14]

Some medical research "payoffs" are demonstrable. Infectious diseases which formerly plagued millions are now virtually unknown. Tuberculosis has not been completely "stamped out," but deaths resulting from the disease have declined to minimal levels; continuing improvement of anti-TB drugs, and wider use of them, caused the death rate from the disease to fall by 31 percent between 1963 and 1967. Deaths from pneumonia have fallen off by 20 percent in the same period.

Although the cause of rheumatoid arthritis has not been finally pinpointed, its crippling effects can now often be prevented thanks to improved methods of diagnosis, recently developed drugs, and more effective methods of physical therapy. Juvenile diabetes was once almost certainly fatal; new biomedical knowledge has now moved us to the position of being able to control this disease so that its victims can lead relatively normal lives, though they still cannot expect to live as long as those without the affliction. In the past decade, important advances have been made in surgery for serious digestive diseases like peptic ulcer and ulcerative colitis; the virus responsible for serum hepatitis has been identified and that disease is being reduced; and prevention and treatment or refractory bleeding in hemophilia has become possible.

Kidney disease has been brought closer to control in the last decade than seemed possible to medical science a generation ago. Kidney infections that used to have a "grave prognosis" can now be effectively treated with drugs. For patients with irreversible kidney failure, the new treatment methods of dialysis and kidney transplantation have proved to be life-savers.

Cataract surgery is no longer the dangerous and uncertain medical treatment it was only a short time ago. Corneal transplants are now more than 50 percent successful, whereas the success rate was only 10 percent two decades ago. And success rates in surgery for detached retinas have climbed from 50 to 90 percent in recent years. Retrolental fibroplasia, which once blinded premature babies, and which so concerned John Fogarty 20 years ago, has been virtually eliminated—in large measure because of the expanded research program which the policy makers and scientist-administrators together decided must be immediately undertaken.

German measles, which affects mothers and children, and Parkinson's disease, which for so long has plagued many older persons, have both been brought under control in recent years. And knowledge about sickle cell anemia, which strikes at

Blacks, has reached the stage where scientists believe it can soon be ameliorated. Even ancient annoyances and embarrassments like goiter, gout, and some forms of deafness can now be controlled, according to NIH officials.

Many would agree with the assertion that "advances in treatment of the mentally and emotionally ill have been revolutionary." [15] Largely through treatment with recently developed drugs, the number of patients in state mental hospitals was reduced by 100,000 between 1960 and 1970. Phenothiazine drugs are now used to control the symptoms of schizophrenia; antidepressants have replaced electroshock as a means of treating depression; and lithium has become a primary and effective agent against manic-depressive psychosis. Mental and emotional illness is still with us, of course. But new drugs and additional numbers of trained (and better dispersed) manpower—reflecting the sizable training programs of the National Institute of Mental Health that have been especially pushed by Congress in the last two decades—mean that far better treatment is more easily accessible and that more persons suffering mental and emotional disorders can now lead what are nearly normal lives.

Dr. Michael DeBakey has claimed the following advances in heart disease treatment alone:

In cardiovascular diseases, more progress has occurred in the past 15 years than in all previously recorded history, owing almost exclusively to laboratory research. Impressive reductions have occurred in the death rate for hypertension, rheumatic heart disease, and stroke. The artificial heart-lung machine, a product of the research laboratory, is now used daily in operating rooms around the country to support blood circulation while surgeons repair diseased hearts or segments of the circulatory system in patients who would previously have been doomed to death.[16]

Indeed, it is now said that "there remain few congenital malformations of the heart that are neither curable nor alleviated by reconstructive surgery." [17]

The importance of the combination of advances in basic knowledge and in clinical practice is strikingly suggested in the area of heart research. Progress in understanding some of the basic biochemical and metabolic controls of the circulatory system has permitted the identification of control points; this in turn has allowed the development of new drugs that can alter such control mechanisms, hence regulate various circulatory ailments. Progress in heart disease and related maladies suggests that "cures" and "controls" do not have to wait until "causes" are fully uncovered. For example, the National Institutes of Health report that "the cause of most hypertension remains a mystery," but that treatment for "nearly all forms of hypertension have become much more practical, predictable, and effective" in the last two decades.[18] Treatment is so effective, in fact, that from the time antihypertension drugs first began to be used in 1952 the death rate from hypertensive heart disease had seen a decline of 59 percent in 1968. New findings showing the effectiveness of drug use in treating moderate hypertension, especially the work of Dr. Edward D. Freis of the Veterans Administration (winner of the Lasker Clinical Research Award in 1971), suggest that the rate will fall still further.

The war against cancer is assessed by some medical doctors and laboratory scientists as going well, but is considered by others to be bogged down in a lack of basic knowledge. Forty years ago the survival rate for cancer victims was only one out of five. Today, using new techniques and new knowledge in radiotherapy, surgery, chemotherapy, and virology, the survival rate is said to be more than one out of three cancer cases, or 40 percent.[19] "Cure," however, means only that the patient is still alive after five years.

Children discovered to have acute leukemia now may live to

almost three years after diagnosis, contrasted with the several months survival period of 1945, thanks to new forms of chemotherapy; 50 percent of patients with Hodgkin's disease, a cancer of the lymph nodes, can now be cured by radiotherapy; and 40 percent of women with breast cancer today are fully cured by applications of new methods of detection and treatment, a percentage significantly above that of the early postwar years. It is estimated that approximately 1.5 million Americans who have had a major form of cancer are leading normal lives.[20]

The National Cancer Institute reports that 37 drugs, many developed in part with NIH funds, can cause temporary remission in 21 different types of cancer which account for about 15 percent of all occurrences of the disease. In some forms of cancer where the rate of tumor cell proliferation is rapid—such as choriocarcinoma and Burkiet's lymphoma—as many as 70 percent of all patients in some studies appear to have been cured.[21] Other cancer forms respond less well to chemotherapy.

The results of the major research and clinical testing effort in chemotherapy, pushed from an early date by some of the medical research lobbyists and their friends in Congress and, at first, somewhat resisted by NIH officials, are judged, in 1971, by the agency as being "dramatic if limited."[22] The critical problem still to be solved in chemotherapy as a means of treatment of fast-growing tumors is how to avoid the destruction of normal cells by the drug agent that is destroying the tumor cells, for the drugs now available destroy both. In other forms of cancer, however, such as acute lymphatic leukemia, the tumor cells are more numerous than the normal cells; so the effect of the drugs against the tumor cells is quantitatively much greater. Under optimal conditions, normal cells can develop out of remaining stem cells after all tumor cells are eliminated. Greater problems remain to be solved in the chemotherapeutic approach to slower-growing tumors, which are not so susceptible to drug treatment and which comprise 85 percent of cancers.

Meanwhile, research in virology continues to hold out hope

for discovery of specific cancer viruses. On December 5, 1971, researchers on the east and west coasts jointly announced discoveries linking an isolated virus with human cancer in humans, moving beyond the long-known fact that viruses can cause cancer in animals. As the *New York Times* commented the following day: "When and if such a link is proved, it is expected to have a profound effect on man's understanding of cancer and, potentially, his ability to deal with it" (p. 13).

Promises of progress toward disease cures, especially cancer cures, continue to titillate us as we read about them in the daily press. Yet a review of the public statements of doctors and scientists and health bureaucrats reveals that some of these promises were offered 20 years ago, with only a little progress having been made in the interim in terms of reducing human affliction. Indeed, most advances in biomedical science, as they have been repetitively described before congressional committees for the last two decades, seem painfully slow. Still, two decades is a very short time, and the usual slow pace of research progress has occasionally been interrupted by a visible, and sometimes dramatic, forward movement resulting in a practical medical ability to control, if not cure, a given disease.

There seems to be an important new element in the reaction to the continuing stream of promises of progress. As the decade of the 1970's unfolds, a sizable body of scientists seems to have joined the politicians and bureaucrats and an eternally hopeful people in believing that medical breakthroughs may occur soon on a variety of fronts. What particularly excites the scientists are the recent advances in basic biomedical knowledge.

Specifically, what is called the "cracking of the genetic code," a very recent accomplishment, is seen as a giant step forward in science, with profound implications for health. In 1970 alone, scientists performed in rapid succession the critical steps of isolating one of those "fundamental units of inheritance" and then synthesizing a gene in the laboratory, experimenting in "genetic surgery" and "genetic therapy." [23] Inherited illness may soon be amenable to correction.[24]

In November 1970 it was reported that "the secret of the hormone that makes bones strong or weak has been deciphered." [25] And one research finding in the same year gave hope that the common cold might yet be scientifically shaken off. The protein which in concentrated form produced "a limited success" in a research project conducted at the National Institute of Allergy and Infectious Diseases was not, the performing scientists warned, "ready to go on the druggists' shelves." But the research team has hopes of developing a better chemical or a better way to give the same chemical to patients which will be more successful.[26]

The detailed understanding gained in the last two decades about fundamental matters—about the structure and functions of cells, hormones, molecules, enzymes—amounts to a virtual explosion of knowledge. It may be in part because basic knowledge has expanded so rapidly that progress in clinical application of disease cures seems to some not to be keeping pace.

The National Institutes of Health have clearly been a major reason for much of the advance in basic knowledge and have contributed singularly important clinical cures. NIH funds were used to make cortisone available for clinical trials in 1948, and the result was the proof of its effectiveness against arthritis and various allergies. The rubella vaccine which reduced the gravity of German measles was developed by the Division of Biologic Standards in 1968 and 1969. NIH funds supported the ultimately successful search for antihypertension drugs and the development of new techniques of heart and vascular surgery. Most of the cancer-chemotherapy drugs were the result of programs of the National Cancer Institute.

Other major clinical advances have come out of research efforts supported by other agencies, both public and private. Isoniazid, a relatively nontoxic drug which has helped bring the death rate from tuberculosis to a minimal level, was initially developed with local funds in New York. The original research which led to the polio vaccines was funded by the National Foundation for Infantile Paralysis; later, at the insistence of Congress and particularly Senator Hill, the Department of Health, Education and Welfare invested in the development and distribution of the vaccine. L-DOPA, the agent so effective against Parkinson's disease, was developed under the auspices of the Atomic Energy Commission. Recent advances in hypertension reduction have come about as a result of ongoing research programs of the Veterans Administration. Private drug houses have led the way in developing tranquilizing drugs.

Often the government's principal health science agency, NIH, has cooperated with other federal or public and private agencies, and the clinical advances have been supported in initial joint efforts, or in tandem with NIH picking up the development of a technique or a drug first supported by another source. Meanwhile, the agency has unquestionably been involved in basic research advances, just as its directorate has wanted, planned, and expected it to be.

What seems closer to attainment in 1972 than ever before is a critical mass of fundamental scientific information based on which disease cures in some areas may now aggressively be sought. This imminent attainment is what has set off a lively new round of activity in the political and public relations arenas as well as in the scientific laboratories. In turn, the newly generated political pressures, accompanying the felt scientific movement, are further encouraging the science bureaucrats to make specific plans for structured efforts at medical advance. Thus, the national medical research enterprise seems to be inching along steadily toward the ultimate goal.

Medical Research and Medical Education

There is also the question whether federal medical research policy, including its component of training new scientists, has had, as Congress has hoped, "a profound though indirect effect upon the education process in our schools that train our physicians, dentists, and other health professionals." The answer is an unqualified yes, but it is not an unqualifiedly happy answer.

Medical school budgets, fed by federal research and related programs, have increased by great magnitudes in the past two decades.[27] Aware of that phenomenon, some officials—both of the giving government and the receiving institutions—have apparently believed that, absent clear-cut federal support for medical education, national research policy has philosophically encompassed and federal research dollars have financially accommodated that function.

Most of those involved in the process of medical and biomedical education believe that the quality of that education has advanced significantly. Boisfeullet Jones, former Vice President for Health Affairs of Emory University, said in his report to Senator Hill's health appropriations subcommittee in 1960 that "the impact of the Federal Program in support of medical teaching has been extremely beneficial and has been largely responsible for an improvement in standards of medical training." [28]

Dr. Thomas B. Turner, while Dean of the Johns Hopkins Medical School, convinced the AMA's Whittaker Commission of "teaching enrichment" from medical research programs. He further pointed out that, within a 15-year period (1951–1966) the number of full-time medical faculty had increased from about 3,500 to over 17,000.[29] That this dramatic increase is largely the result of federal medical research and training expenditures is perhaps shown more clearly by the statistic that, by 1970, fully one-half the total medical faculty of the country received at least part of their salaries from federal sources.

Growth, however, does not inevitably result in strength, and what is good for the country is not necessarily good for given institutions.

With federal research and related funds, the medical schools of Harvard, Case Western, Baylor, Alabama, and Pennsylvania, over the last twenty years, have increased their full-time medical faculties by numbers roughly averaging some 200 percent. Yet the number of students enrolled in courses of study leading to the M.D. degree has increased only marginally between the early 1950's and 1970: by 16 percent at Harvard, 5 percent at Baylor, 12 percent at Case Western. At Alabama, in Senator Hill's home state, the number of M.D. candidates has increased significantly, going from 219 in 1950 to 348 in 1970, an increase of 59 percent. But at most medical schools it appears that the minimally increased enrollments of students training to become medical doctors probably would have occurred without federal research funds for most of this period. Meanwhile, medical schools were in as severe, or more severe, trouble in 1971 as they were in 1949 and 1950.

Those who have assumed that there was a third goal implicit in national medical research policy—that in addition to the reduction of disease effects and the creation of a great national medical research network, the policy was also expected if not designed to support medical education—would have to rate the policy unsuccessful on that score. But the support of medical education broadly, including the production of doctors, has never been a solid, explicit component of medical research policy. Nor has support of medical schools per se.

Twenty years ago (in 1949 and again in 1951) the Congress specifically rejected a proposal for federal support of medical schools by means of institutional grants, and of medical students by means of scholarships and loans. There was universal acknowledgment of the financial plight of medical schools. Albert Lasker testified, on the basis of personal contact with "the heads of the greatest medical schools in the United States," that they were "on the verge of financial catastrophe." [30] Dr. Alan Gregg, Director of Medical Sciences for the Rockefeller Foundation, warned: "Unless our medical schools receive substantially larger sums for their essential expenses, we shall not in the future have the care which modern medicine could provide." [31]

Though everyone recognized the institutions' financial trouble, some doubted the need for more doctors. Dr. Louis H. Bauer, chairman of the AMA's Board of Trustees, told the Senate that, while the country needed more doctors, "we are getting them steadily." Besides, he added, "you must remember that illness is diminishing." Furthermore, the proposal to support medical schools with federal funds "would give the Government a foot in the door—in fact, probably two feet in the door—for federal control of medical education." [32]

The ultimate refusal of Congress, at the end of the two-year fight from 1949 to 1951 to provide a direct solution to the problem of adequate financing for medical education, did not cause that problem to go away. Everyone recognized that medical schools were in trouble; almost everyone believed that the predicted shortage of physicians would occur and would have an adverse impact on the nation's health; and some still thought the federal government was duty-bound to help.

In December 1952, as he prepared to leave office, President Truman received the report of the President's Commission on the Health Needs of the Nation. The Commission was chaired by Dr. Paul B. Magnuson, a prominent physician, known Republican, and accepted objective analyst. After two years of study, Dr. Magnuson predicted a serious physician shortage ranging from 22,000 to 45,000. Specifically, projecting a population of 171 million people in the United States by 1960, the report stated: "To bring the regions of the Nation with the present lowest ratios of physicians to population up to the current average for the nation would require 22,000 more physicians by 1960 than the predicted supply by that year. This might be considered a minimum estimate of need." As part of the solution, the Commission recommended the provision of federal funds to schools of medicine, dentistry, nursing, and public health for facilities, operating funds, and student support including "federal scholarships to students who could not otherwise attend schools for education and training in the health professions." [33]

Three more reports of distinguished professional and lay people would echo the same general needs in the late 1950's: the Bayne-Jones Report in 1958,[34] the Bayne Report in 1959,[35] and the Jones Report in 1960. But there was to be no action in direct response to that need, no national policy to meet the national condition, for yet a while. Nor was there any indication that the Congress had tacitly changed its position on federal aid to medical education. The Fogarty committee warned the National Institutes of Health in 1957 that funds for medical research were not to be spent for broad support of medical schools and medical education: "The Committee does not doubt that most medical schools need some additional financial assistance, however, funds appropriated to the National Institutes of Health are not for the purpose of general assistance to medical schools." [36]

In 1963, with the enactment of the Health Professions Educational Assistance Act, Congress took a first, small step toward providing direct support for medical and paramedical education.[37] Such support was limited to grants for facilities construction and student loans. The authority of that legislation was broadened in 1965 and 1966, and a more comprehensive means of federal support was provided in the Health Manpower Act of 1968.[38] Under these authorities, a total of over $1.3 billion has been appropriated, from fiscal 1963 through fiscal 1971, for direct support of medical schools and allied health professional schools. In the same period over $5.2 billion was appropriated for extramural research grants. In 1968 the Bureau of Health Professions Education and Manpower Training of the Department of Health, Education and Welfare was placed in the National Institutes of Health. In 1970 it was designated the Bureau of Health Manpower Education. Recent programs of that Bureau have begun to affect the numbers of students in the health professions that institutions are able and willing to enroll.

Even with such new efforts, now placed in direct relation to medical research by organizational rearrangements, the impact on medical education has remained slight. One reason is that the new programs have not received appropriations anywhere close to their authorization levels, from 1969 through 1971 remaining roughly $100 million less per year than the ceiling authorized. Limitation on program scope and paucity of funds in the federal plan has directly affected the production of doctors, in that, as the National Academy of Sciences points out: "In contrast to graduate students and postdoctoral fellows, virtually all of whom receive financial support from some source, by and large it is still necessary for the families of medical students to provide the funds necessary for their maintenance and tuition during their medical education.[39]

Meanwhile, there has been a direct governmental mandate, all along, to produce additional medical researchers. To train them would cost institutions money, and so with governmental approval the Heart, Cancer, and Mental Health Institutes in the early 1950's began allowing faculty salaries to be included in the costs of training grants. By fiscal 1960, about $125 million of the NIH budget—about one-fourth of its total appropriation of $430 million, and one-half of its budget for extramural research grants—was being spent for training grants and fellowships. Growth of those programs continued, but the proportionate increase did not. In 1970 approximately $200 million was being spent for training grants and fellowships; that represented approximately one-seventh of the total NIH appropriation, but over one-third of its extramural grant appropriation.[40]

It has not been the broad growth trends, but the emphasis on training medical researchers and granting allowances for faculty salaries for the purpose that has led some people to believe that the financial problems of medical schools, and perhaps the need for more practicing physicians, would be taken care of. But the NIH directorate has been fastidious about what the training funds are and are not to be spent for. Congressional rejection of direct support of medical schools and the training of physicians throughout most of the past 20 years has been, in a way, a more explicit policy guide than congressional desire for cure of dread disease. The latter policy goal permitted various approaches, hence some managerial latitude, but the former was believed to be absolutely binding. While Dr. Shannon always preferred a broad interpretation of congressional purpose, he would not be a party to outright subversion.

Hence, although the output of M.D.'s increased relatively slightly from 1950 to 1970, the production of biomedical research scientists increased markedly. The number of students at Harvard Medical School seeking the M.D. degree increased by 16 percent, going from 502 in 1950 to 583 in 1970; but the number of Ph.D. students rose from 50 to 171 in the same period, a 240 percent increase. The medical faculty, of course, taught both groups. Case Western Reserve Medical School's M.D. student population rose from 323 to 364 between 1950 and 1970, while the number of its Ph.D. students rose from 0 to 132. At the University of Pennsylvania Medical School, the M.D. student population increased by only 8 percent from 1960 to 1970, but the Ph.D. student group increased by 80 percent. Alabama and Baylor Medical Schools had no students seeking the Ph.D. degree in 1950; in 1970 they had 150 and 99 respectively.

Nationwide, the National Academy of Sciences reported that, for the academic year 1968–69, "medical students constituted less than half the total educational responsibilities" of medical schools and their teaching faculties.[41]

In short, federal research and training funds going into medical schools have followed rather precisely the purposes originally stated: they have supported biomedical research, and they have supported the training of great numbers of additional researchers. Federal research funds have not supported medical schools per se. Instead, the federal government has used medical schools and other institutions to support those functions essential to the central research policy goals.

Congress may have generally felt, as key Congressmen certainly wished, that there would be beneficial fallout for medical education from medical research policies and programs. But, as has been suggested, the mere enunciation of policy goals does not produce policy. Whatever else is involved, 1) clear statement of purpose, 2) a working consensus to achieve it, 3) agreement on means as well as ends, and 4) continuing, focused fiscal support of integral programs are four ingredients which are essential to real policy. None of those elements has obtained, in the last two decades, in the matter of benefits expected to accrue to medical education from medical research.

When the flow of medical research funds leveled off, medical school deans and other university officials increased their efforts to get federal policy makers to consider new approaches. They admitted that research funds had sometimes been sought for broad institutional purposes, in a sort of "bootleg operation." [42] But they suggested that the policy makers invited that situation by their longtime infatuation with research and their persistent refusal to offer other substantial mechanisms and funds to support other functions of their institutions—like teaching—which were essential to the overall viability of the institutions, hence to medical research as well.

In February 1971, President Nixon presented a broad health plan to Congress in which he proposed several ways to increase the production of medical and allied health personnel. Congressional leaders were likewise willing to take the final step at last. In November 1971, the Comprehensive Health Manpower Act of 1971 not only authorized direct federal support of medical education, through capitation grants, but offered financial incentives to those medical schools that would increase their enrollments of medical, dental, and nursing students and additional incentives to those that would do so by shortening their curricula.[43]

The major architect of the new federal approach was Congressman Paul G. Rogers (D., Fla.), chairman of the Subcommittee on Public Health and Environment of the House Committee on Interstate and Foreign Commerce. Senator Edward Kennedy (D., Mass.) led the effort on the Senate side. Both men had been moving toward positions of leadership in health matters, in part because earlier committee assignments and legislative involvements had spurred their interest and in part because they recognized, as did the President, that "health" was developing as a major concern of the the people, potentially affecting elections. Helping them to that realization was an important new lobbying force (if not-so-new organization), the Association of American Medical Colleges. Representing the institutions that had been the keystones in the national medical research network and the direct beneficiaries of research funds, the AAMC was finally vigorously asserting its interests, and was doing so successfully. Nor did it confine itself to new medical education issues, for it plunged into a battle over proposed creation of a new agency that would be assigned the job of conquering cancer. Members of the old medical research lobby were surprised at the strength the new lobby seemed to possess.

The Integration of Medical Research and Other Health Programs

Clearly the federal government's new health thrusts in the recent years comprise a more balanced approach to the health needs of the nation than its earlier primary reliance on medical research, hospital construction, and public health programs. That approach will be even more balanced and comprehensive if other fronts are opened in the near future. This is likely, for the ingredients exist to produce national concern, and deep, widespread national concerns usually produce political action.

Medical research has enjoyed long popularity because it has been perceived as a weapon against a threat that is at once personal and national: dread disease. Similarly, spending for research and development programs in defense, space, and areas related to national security reached their peak during the continuance of the cold war, for "R & D" was expected to produce potent answers to the potential threat to our collective security.

As the 1970's unfold, the high costs of health care for all citizens, the continuing unavailability to some citizens of any medical care, the failure of the "health system" to alleviate chronic national health problems, to reduce morbidity and mortality rates among various groups—all combine to constitute what has been labeled a "health crisis," a situation perceived by ever growing numbers of citizens as a national threat which is, once more, both collective and personal. It is the kind of situation which not only demands action, but which will produce popular support for whatever reasonable, comprehensive action is taken. Politicians, especially elected officials, know this, and that is why 1971 produced new federal health initiatives and why the coming years will produce still more.

As in the 1940's, the major battle is over national health insurance. Only this time, odds are heavily in favor of the enactment of some plan. One clue in that regard is that more than half of the members of the House of Representatives have each introduced some measure designed to expand health insurance coverage to more American citizens.

The old alliance of the forties—organized labor, key liberal Senators, and Mrs. Albert Lasker—has reappeared, reinvigorated. Its new plan is not dissimilar from the old one; introduced by Edward Kennedy and fourteen other Senators, it proposes comprehensive health insurance coverage for most citizens. The cost of the plan is unclear; but Senator Kennedy has stated that if the plan had been in effect in 1970, it would have covered 70 percent of total expenditures for health care, in the amount of $41 billion.[44]

The Nixon Administration is responding with a more limited approach, but even that response stands out in contrast with the adamant refusal of conservative forces of earlier decades to admit the need for *some* program requiring *some* government subsidy. The Nixon plan would mainly cover the poor and near poor.

The American Medical Association is seeking a new image, and may even be coming into a new posture. It has now cancelled its self-supported medical research effort and ceased to tout its ability to secure enough funds to provide scholarships and loans to all medical students who need them. Although the organization still spends an enormous part of its budget and of its official deliberations on public relations, it has finally agreed that federal support of medical research is good; that there is a doctor shortage; and that federal aid for medical education is necessary. Further, it has proposed that the medical profession itself inaugurate efforts to insure that the poor do not go without medical service, and that the profession should further "innovate" by such means as group practice. The AMA will very possibly support the Nixon health insurance plan, and may do so in part out of conviction about its merits as well as out of fear of more expansive alternatives.

The private health insurance industry may be the liberals' villain in the battle shaping up. But like the AMA, that industry seems to recognize that federally subsidized medical insurance for a large number of American citizens is bound to come; for rather than mobilizing to oppose any such plan, they have instead been working with the Administration on draft legislation.

Federal support of medical education is now a reality. Thus, when some form of national health insurance becomes law, the comprehensive health program for the nation proposed by President Harry S Truman in 1946 will finally have come into being.

That a single vested-interest organization, the American Medical Association, successfully thwarted for so long the effectuation of that plan has been documented. But although this fact is important to this story of national policy evolution, it should not be overemphasized. For rarely in our democracy has any broad government plan that is aimed at promoting the general welfare, or specific components of it like the people's health, been swiftly adopted according to such a grand design as that laid out by President Truman a quarter of a century ago.

Meanwhile, federal biomedical research and related programs have carried a heavy burden over the last 25 years. Unaccompanied by the real thing, medical research has *had* to serve as "national health insurance." Lacking a comprehensive system for the delivery of existing health knowledge and health care techniques to all persons specifically in need, the country has seemed to expect that new results of medical research, and the expanding presence of a research enterprise in medical schools and university science departments and hospitals, would suffice, following a kind of "trickle-down" theory, to produce better health for the American people generally. Many persons, hanging onto the occasional congressional mention of a policy by-product of "institutional stability," have thought that health research funds might, alone, serve the health of institutions of higher education.

Such expectations no longer ride the back of national medical research policy; but the central goal—conquering dread disease—has become even more pronounced.

XII   Conquering Cancer: Renewing the Goal

Aroused demands for more direct approaches to various national health needs have not lessened interest in the goal Matthew Neely first sought in 1927 and Mary Lasker has continued to push since 1942. On the contrary, the popular demand for a scientific victory over cancer has become more intense.

In the spring of 1970, Senator Ralph Yarborough, chairman of the Senate Labor and Public Welfare Committee, appointed a Committee of Consultants on Cancer consisting of 13 medical scientists and 13 laymen. Yarborough stated two primary tasks of the Committee: to examine the adequacy of present support of cancer research, and "to recommend to Congress and to the American people what must be done to achieve cures for the major forms of cancer by 1976—the 200th anniversary of the founding of this great Republic." Cancer, said the Senator from Texas, is "a vicious disease" and "mankind's most relentless foe." He urged new efforts to guarantee "that the conquest of cancer become a highly visible national goal." [1]

Like his predecessors who had espoused the cause of medical research generally, or particular medical research causes, Ralph Yarborough was genuinely concerned about what appeared to be a lag in the fight against cancer. In the three years preceding the establishment of the special cancer panel, the budget of the National Cancer Institute, said Yarborough, "had been barely sufficient to maintain the status quo." [2] Also like his predecessors, the Senator surely hoped that the Committee of Consultants' endeavors, in addition to bolstering the fight against cancer, would bolster his chances of re-election. In the end, Yarborough's espousal of a popular national research cause was no more helpful to him politically than similar efforts had been to Neely in 1928 or Joseph Ransdell in 1930. Yarborough was defeated in the Texas Democratic primary in the summer of 1970. For the last six months of his senatorial career he gave high priority to his Committee's Cancer Panel, as it came to be known.

Mary Lasker, inveterate strategist of the medical research lobby, and Dr. Sidney Farber, visionary veteran in the scientific search for answers to cancer, had proposed the Committee of Consultants to Senator Yarborough. The committee-commission approach was one that had served well in the past; it had worked particularly well in 1959–60, when Senate health leaders had needed outside professional endorsement of their efforts to get a less than enthusiastic Republican administration to go along with their plan for greatly increased biomedical research funds. The political scene in 1970 being quite similar to that of 1960, Mrs. Lasker, Dr. Farber, and Senator Yarborough reasoned that a new outside, nonpartisan group could give professional, objective advice that would be persuasive to members of Congress and, possibly, to key decision makers in the executve branch.

Naturally, the members of the cancer panel were not to be randomly chosen. They would of course include both laymen and medical scientists, and both Democrats and Republicans. But they especially were to include known friends. Senator Yarborough consulted with his ranking counterpart on the Labor and Public Welfare Committee, Senator Jacob Javits (R., N.Y.) about possible appointments to the cancer panel, but he principally relied on a list suggested by Mrs. Lasker. Of the 26 persons named to the panel, a number of them were her experienced allies: Elmer Bobst and Emerson Foote had been partners in the effort to reform the American Cancer Society in the early 1940's; Anna Rosenberg Hoffman had opened doors to the White House in the Roosevelt Administration; Dr. Mathilde Krim's husband, Arthur, had been a fellow fund-raiser for various Democratic candidates including Lyndon Johnson; I. W. Abel of the United Steel Workers was carrying on labor's part of the alliance that had, since the 1940's, sought the enactment of national health insurance; William McCormick Blair was a close personal friend; and Dr. Solomon Garb, through his small book of 1968, *Cure for Cancer: A National Goal*, had helped convince Mrs. Lasker of the possibility of the ultimate conquest of cancer. The Rockefeller family's longtime interest in medical research was renewed with Laurance Rockefeller's appointment to the Committee. Designated chairman of the panel was Benno C. Schmidt, managing partner of J. H. Whitney & Company, member of the board of the Sloan-Kettering Foundation, independent Republican, native Texan, and friend of Senator Javits. Dr. Farber was named vice chairman.

Naturally, Col. Luke Quinn and Mike Gorman were to be behind-the-scenes advisers in the effort, though they steered clear of one another. NIH officials had little if anything to say about the creation of the Committee of Consultants, but when it was a fact of life the National Cancer Institute offered logistical help and even lent personnel to assist in the day-to-day activities of the panel and in writing its report. Florence Mahoney, having already launched a new special crusade of her own—the creation of an institute for research on aging—was unavailable to help on the cancer effort. Some of Mrs. Lasker's friends and some of her critics thought the approach, and even the subject, were awfully old hat. When Senator Yarborough was defeated, most were sure the new cause would go nowhere.

In December 1970 the Committee of Consultants submitted their report to Yarborough, a few days before he was to leave the Senate. Their recommendations were predictable. They urged an all-out attack on "the implacable foe," requiring the expenditure of hundreds of millions of dollars annually, and they recommended the creation of a new National Cancer Authority.[3] Based on an assessment of recent research progress and present research potential, an assessment of continuing human need and persistent human fear (and, though its report failed to specify it, an assessment that the existing organization was unable or unwilling to mount a successful, final assault on the disease), the Committee of Consultants proposed, as it were, the solution that Matthew Neely had proposed in the House of Representatives in 1946.

The existence of continuing popular concern about cancer was no less real because the old research lobby's hand was much in the works of the cancer panel. As the consultants pointed out, "a poll taken in 1966 showed that 62 percent of the public feared cancer more than any other disease." That is an understandable fear, the Committee suggested because, "of the 200 million Americans alive today, 50 million will die of cancer." [4] And for once, a number of respectable scientists and science administrators (including directors and former directors of institutes of NIH) genuinely believed that progress in basic knowledge rendered a new, targeted attack on cancer practicable and desirable. It is not surprising that political interest followed closely on the heels of popular concern and professional assessments of scientific feasibility.

The House of Representatives in 1970 also passed a resolution calling for a national crusade against cancer.[5] The Nixon Administration in the preceding two years had increased funds for cancer research in the NIH budget while holding steady, if not decreasing, funds for many other research fields. Immediately after the Committee of Consultants released its report, Senator Edward Kennedy announced his intention to push for legislation to implement its recommendations when the new Congress convened in 1971.

If the Cancer Consultants' recommendations were no surprise to those who had followed the research lobby's work over the years, the reaction of the National Institutes of Health to the "new plan" was just as perfect in its predictability. "I'm against it," said Robert Q. Marston, Director of NIH. The cancer research budget of NIH, he said, was continuing to rise; and to separate cancer research "from interplay from other research in the diseases of man" would be wasteful and wrong.[6]

There was, indeed, only one real surprise in the new version of a very old scenario. The President of the United States personally reopened the budget of the National Institutes of Health in early January 1971—to the particular amazement of the NIH directorate—and added to the figure his lieutenants had set an extra $100 million for "an intensive campaign to find a cure for cancer." [7]

It was natural that Ted Kennedy take Ralph Yarborough's place in this effort. All the Kennedy brothers had served on the Labor and Public Welfare Committee, and Ted had become increasingly interested in health matters, which had become increasingly important political issues. It was also natural for Kennedy to take up Mrs. Lasker's cause. She had been supportive of his brother, the late President; and as soon as her friend Lyndon Johnson had announced his decision not to run for re-election in 1968, she had immediately endorsed the candidacy of her Senator, Robert Kennedy of New York.

It was natural, as well, that Edward Kennedy's announced sponsorship of the cancer panel recommendations made Richard Nixon look more closely at the issues involved. Some of the President's advisers had been concerned about the effects of declining (if only by virtue of inflation) federal support of research in universities and other academic institutions. The President's Science Advisers, first Dr. Lee DuBridge and subsequently Dr. Edward David, Jr., had helped secure additional funds for the National Science Foundation. George Schultz, the director of the federal budget who had come to the Nixon Administration first as Secretary of Labor from the University of Chicago, was a man with a scholar's understanding of the importance of research—and an economist's appreciation of productivity. It was, nonetheless, after Kennedy's public declaration that he was going to try to secure congressional approval of a new "conquest of cancer" effort that an inquiry was made among presidential aides as to which medical research areas might, with additional funds, prompt practical results and whether, in particular, cancer might be one of those areas.

On January 21, the President launched his own cancer initiative in the course of his State of the Union address. He did so in language that must have appealed to the nonscientist supporters of medical research but undoubtedly offended scientific purists. (It also made some of his own advisors nervous.) Said the President: "The time has come when the same kind of concentrated effort that split the atom and took man to the moon should be turned toward conquering this dread disease. Let us make a total commitment to achieve this goal." [8]

A few days later, on January 29, Senator Kennedy introduced, for himself and Senator Javits, the Conquest of Cancer Act— identical to the act Senator Yarborough had proposed to implement the recommendations of the cancer panel.[9] The bill called for the establishment of a new national cancer authority, with an administrator and several assistant administrators to be appointed by the President with the advice and consent of the Senate. The administrator and his deputy would serve a five-year term and would submit annual reports to the President on progress made toward the goal. A national Cancer Advisory Board would be created, comprised of nine scientists and nine laymen—the equal division that Mrs. Lasker had found to be very important. The National Cancer Institute would be absorbed by the National Cancer Authority, with the Cancer Advisory Board replacing the existing National Advisory Cancer Council with its lesser number of lay members.

Following the unusual if salutary precedent set in 1948 when open-ended authorization of funds were approved for all the National Institutes of Health, the bill read: "For purposes of carrying out any of the programs, functions, or activities authorized by this Act, there are authorized to be appropriated for each fiscal year such sums as may be necessary." [10] (The Committee of Consultants had recommended a beginning annual appropriation of $400 million, with subsequent annual appropriations to reach a level of $1 billion by 1976.)

When the Senate committee commenced its hearings in

March of 1971, the Nixon Administration still had not spelled out the details of its plans for an enlarged attack on cancer. All that was known about the President's intentions was that he expected NIH and its Cancer Institute to continue to oversee the effort and that he had himself suggested the possibility of open-ended funding. He had said that, in addition to the extra $100 million he had added to the cancer research budget for that year, he would make available additional funds as needed to take advantage of any new scientific leads that held promise of a "breakthrough."

Science Adviser Edward David, Jr., underscored the Administration's plan to have the new effort remain within NIH. In his speech to the Association of American Medical Colleges in February 1971, Dr. David said: "It is the President's belief that having honed and sharpened our biomedical research mechanism, the National Institutes of Health, we should now use it and call upon it as we embark upon this new adventure." He also suggested that scientists and science spokesmen within the Administration were still trying to keep the political impulses, and their rhetorical expression, in check. In structuring the new approach, said David, "we must take account of the differences between this effort and the Apollo and Manhattan projects. In cancer, we do not know whether the critical experiment has yet been done . . . This aspect presents a stark contrast with Apollo and nuclear energy. Indeed we do not believe in an AEC or NASA for cancer." [11]

While pressing on with his own plan, Senator Kennedy pressed the Administration to reveal the components of its announced new thrust. Following the first round of hearings in early March, Kennedy asked for and received from Secretary of Health, Education and Welfare Elliot L. Richardson—who had first had to deal with congressional boosters of medical research in the later Eisenhower years when he was Arthur Flemming's Assistant Secretary—a description of the President's plan. According to Secretary Richardson's letter of April 2, 1971, the Administration proposed: raising the Cancer Institute to bureau level within NIH; making the director of the bureau a deputy director of NIH; and giving the Cancer Bureau authority over funds for cancer research throughout the National Institutes of Health, regardless of which Institute would expend them.[12] In short, while cancer was raised to a new level of importance and visibility by virtue of additional dollars and a promotion of sorts for the man in charge of cancer research, there were to be no fundamental changes in the organizational arrangement of NIH.

Spokesmen for the Administration, including Dr. Robert Q. Marston, Director of NIH, and Surgeon General Jesse Steinfeld, continued to emphasize that all parties were agreed on the importance of a major new effort to control (if not cure, they added) the dread disease. There was essential unanimity of purpose, they said, complimenting the Senate committee for its concern and willingness.[13] And, they said reassuringly, NIH can and will do the job.

Fundamentally, it was the organizational arrangement that the reinvigorated cancer research lobby thought had to be changed if real progress was to be made. Benno Schmidt repeatedly attacked the present arrangement with its "six layers of bureaucracy": to obtain authority for important decisions, the director of the National Cancer Institute had to go through the Deputy Director of NIH to the Director, who had to go through the Surgeon General of the Public Health Service to the Assistant Secretary of HEW, who had to clear matters with the Secretary. And for that matter, the Secretary might have to clear a given decision with the Director of the Office of Management and Budget, speaking for the President.[14]

But it was bureaucratic attitudes as well as organizational hierarchy that bothered the research lobby. They continued to doubt that the NIH directorate as a whole really wanted to find a cure or series of cures for cancer as fast as possible. Dr. Carl Baker, director of the Cancer Institute, acted and talked very much like the activist leader of a purposeful research activity. For one thing, more and more cancer research money was being spent on contracts aimed at specific research targets, rather than on grants for undifferentiated research. The battle against cancer, Baker suggested, was getting to be "like the Battle of Britain . . . There's no fooling around with committees in wartime. There isn't time. And it's immoral to fiddle around now." [15] But even if they thought of Baker as personally committed, the representatives of the Cancer Panel who testified before Senator Kennedy in favor of their own recommendations thought Baker, or any other Cancer Institute director, was boxed in under present circumstances.

The NIH central directorate smarted under the allegation that bureaucratic attitudes and red-taped processes were retarding the search for answers to cancer and would continue to do so unless the new cancer attack was removed from their supervision. "My colleagues and I have spent much of our lives trying to move the national research enterprise towards productive results," said a senior NIH official, "and it makes me mad for Johnny-come-latelies like Benno Schmidt to go around saying we're just a bunch of bureaucrats who are not committed to finding a cure for cancer." Secretary Richardson expressed doubts about the objectivity of the Schmidt-Lasker panel's investigation of existing organizational arrangements and attitudes, and made remarks permitting the inference that there may have been a little in-house complicity—and even a little empire building—affecting the cancer panel's recommendation of a new agency to conduct the war on cancer. Senator Peter Dominick (R., Colo.) queried Richardson about the cancer panel's charge of bureaucratic inefficiencies and their effect on cancer progress. Richardson wrote in response that except for a brief courtesy call on the director of the National Institutes of Health before their study began, and a visit with him after their recommendations were formulated, members and staff of the cancer panel mainly closeted themselves with officials of the National Cancer Institute. Recounting the history of the panel's "study," Richardson emphasized: "Thus it is clear that, with the exception of officials and employees of the National Cancer Institute, members of the panel did not consult with top management officials either of the Department or the National Institutes of Health with regard to the scientific or managerial aspects of cancer research." [16]

Continuing the long-established tradition, the new congressional medical research leaders were bipartisan in their posture toward the executive branch. Senator Javits was even more emphatic than Senator Kennedy in stating the prevailing attitude. Addressing the Administration witnesses in the March hearings, Javits said:

> Our people suffering with this particular dread disease, somehow or other, I think have a general feeling that this is unnecessary, that we can break through, not in the years it will take the bureaucracy, but with the concentrated, high level project of the character proposed in the Kennedy-Javits bill. Therefore I believe that the likelihood is that, unless you gentlemen have some very good alternative, that the Congress will make the decision. It is not necessary to have the doctors make it, or even the Commission [Committee of Consultants, or National Advisory Cancer Council] make it. The Congress will make it.[17]

As the alternative suggested in Secretary Richardson's letter did not sound very persuasive, the Labor and Public Welfare Committee continued to move toward the adoption of the plan proposed by the Schmidt-Lasker panel and guided along by Kennedy and Javits.

Opposition to the plan was building, but through the spring of 1971 it was ineffectual against the combination of a strong bipartisan Senate team leading the advance (according to a strategy worked out by a distinguished, nonpartisan outside group), buoyed by the always presumed and increasingly vocal mass of citizens who wanted cancer conquered. Robert Marston was more active on the Hill than he had been in his entire three-year period as director of NIH, seizing every opportunity to try to persuade Senators to oppose the Kennedy-Javits bill.[18]

Senator Gaylord Nelson (D., Wisc.) made a diversionary attack by proposing that the whole of NIH be separated from HEW, as an independent health research agency whose director would report to the President. He was supported openly by three scientist members of the Senate cancer panel, Dr. Joshua Lederberg, Dr. Henry S. Kaplan, and Dr. Harold P. Rusch; and he was supported in spirit by many people at NIH.[19]

Dr. James Shannon was physically unable to appear before the Kennedy committee, but his position on the issue was strong, and predictable. Dr. Philip R. Lee, chancellor of the University of California, San Francisco, and former Assistant Secretary for Health of HEW, read a letter from Dr. Shannon into the record in connection with his own testimony opposing the separation of cancer research from NIH auspices. The proposed new cancer authority, Shannon wrote, was "dangerously destructive." Acknowledging the old medical research lobbyists' "invaluable role" in awakening public interest in medical research, and their "positive contribution" in "modulating the scientific judgment" about research directions, Shannon warned against letting the lobby have its way in their desire to isolate the cancer effort in a separate program he feared they would control. If that happened, he said, scientific emphasis "would be entirely determined by uncritical zealots, experts in advertising, and rapacious 'empire builders.'"[20]

Dr. John A. D. Cooper of the Association of American Medical Colleges, assisted by Joseph Murtagh, longtime aide of Dr. Shannon, was developing opposition on behalf of his constituency. That constituency, Dr. Cooper emphasized, included all 103 medical schools in the nation, 401 of the major teaching hospitals, and 47 academic medical societies representing faculties of those and other institutions: in short, "the scientists and institutions which have had much to do with the great progress in medicine which we have witnessed in our lifetime." [21] But neither his nor others' testimony before the Senate committee, or their public utterances elsewhere, seemed to sway the growing group of senatorial "zealots."

On the other side of the fight, Mary Lasker was leaving no stone unturned in what was already looking like the most important victory in her remarkable career. She suggested to her friend Ann Landers, the popular and perennial guidance counselor and social arbiter whose syndicated column appears in 750 newspapers with a total circulation estimated at 54 million, that she help spread the word about the importance of the Conquest of Cancer bill. Miss Landers did so in April, urging her readers to become "part of the mightiest offensive against a single disease in the history of our country." To join that mighty effort one had only to write his Senator. Miss Landers prophetically explained: "If enough citizens let their Senators know they want bill S. 34 [the Kennedy-Javits bill] passed, it will pass." [22]

The response was overwhelming. Senator John Tunney (D., Cal.) estimated that he got approximately 25,000 pieces of mail as a result of the Landers' column.[23] Senator Fred Harris (D., Okla.)—whose earlier exploration of biomedical research as chairman of a subcommittee of the Government Operations Committee had provided him with convictions opposing a separate cancer conquest agency—found the wave of popular opinion building so fast in Oklahoma after Miss Landers' exposition that he decided he could no longer delay joining the front ranks of the "mighty offensive"—especially in an election year when he was already in political trouble. He was one of the last Senators to attach his name to a bill endorsing a new, independent attack on cancer.

The successful attempt to generate wide public support for the Kennedy-Javits bill through the mass media—a technique which had always been one of Florence Mahoney's specialties but the efficacy of which Mary Lasker up until then had doubted —was not the only one used by the cancer lobby. Direct attention continued to be focused on members of the Committee of Consultants on Cancer, and comparisons between medical research and other expenditures, emotional appeals, and challenges to greatness were added to more specifically scientific or organizational reasons why Senators should support the separate cancer authority. Mrs. Anna Rosenberg Hoffman was the last member of the cancer panel and one of the last witnesses to address the Senate Health Subcommittee. She reminded the Senators that, as Assistant Secretary of Defense, she had often come before the Senate and asked for "sums so great that the money we are asking for today for the fight against cancer seems infinitesimal." That experience in the Department of Defense meant, she told the committee, that "I know what it means to be in an agency where you have to go through these bureaucratic procedures and I know what it means to be in an agency that is only responsible to the President and to the Congress." Her final challenge was:

> Senator, you and the members of the U.S. Senate have the opportunity, if I may say so, seldom given in the lives of men—even Senators—to turn on the power that eventually could save the lives of hundreds of thousands of men, women, and children in the United States and pass on that knowledge all over the world, and the name of America would be blessed.
>
> You and I have known some of your ablest colleagues who might have been saved and the many dear ones in our own families who still can be saved if we waste no more time and let S. 34 be our next "man on the moon." [24]

Finishing its hearings in April, and still not having formally received the President's plan, the Senate committee moved toward putting the final touches on its cancer bill.

Kenneth R. Cole, Jr., the White House staff member assigned to coordinate the follow-up to the President's cancer plans, says that the Chief Executive had not focused his attention on details of required organizational changes when he first announced his intentions to step up the attack on cancer.[25] That is no doubt why, from the time President Nixon first addressed the subject in January through completion of the Senate hearings in April, no one was sure what his personal preferences in the matter really were. What was assumed to be the Administration position, and what seemed to be a quite clear position, was spelled out in Secretary Richardson's letter to Senator Kennedy on April 2. That position was to maintain the integrity of the National Institutes of Health, not only keeping the new cancer effort an integral part of that agency but doing so without severely upsetting existing arrangements and existing balance.

The Department of Health, Education and Welfare stuck to that position privately as well as publicly in the month of April, but the final presidential decision in fact had not been made. Even after the Richardson letter had been submitted to the Senate, others continued to press the President to propose a plan more nearly according with the recommendations of the cancer panel.

Elmer Bobst, the President's "foster father," may be the only mutual friend Mary Lasker and Richard Nixon share. If so, one friend proved sufficient for the purpose at hand—especially given the additional means available for impressing the President. Mr. Bobst called President Nixon more than once to urge his support of the tack that Bobst and his colleagues on the panel had recommended. Whether his arguments by themselves were enough to persuade a President is not certain, but a White House staff member acknowledges that "when Mr. Bobst calls, the President gets on the line." Coinciding with Mr. Bobst's calls of April 1971 was a message to the White House from Senator Javits: the Kennedy-Javits bill was going to be reported out of the Labor and Public Welfare Committee, and it had enough support to be passed by the Senate regardless of what the President's formal proposal would look like.

President Nixon perhaps thought he had stolen the march from the congressional anticancer leaders when he made an extra $100 million available for cancer research in January 1971, promising still more money and streamlined organizational arrangements in the battle against the disease. But as in 1937, when the bill to establish the National Cancer Institute was introduced, popular support gave congressional action such momentum that executive response could easily turn out to have been superfluous. The political signs of the moment suggested that the President would have to run to stay ahead of the crusade he wanted to lead.

With his advisers still divided over the proper approach, the President was presented four alternatives for his cancer attack plan during the month of April 1971: 1) To make no changes in the organizational structure of the National Institutes of Health beyond those already suggested by Secretary Richardson, and simply to rely on the new money to produce new results. 2) To separate, by administrative action, the National Institutes of Health from the parent Department of HEW, giving biomedical research greater visibility and greater importance by having a director appointed by and reporting to the President. 3) To request a legislative mandate to accomplish the last objective. 4) To create a new and elevated "conquest of cancer agency" within NIH, whose director would report directly to the Secretary of HEW without going through other officials of NIH or underlings in the Department, and whose budget would similarly escape the oppression of some of the existing layers of bureaucratic control.

Examining those alternatives, the President made a quick decision. He created another alternative, and chose it: focusing on the fourth possibility suggested by his staff, he struck out "the Secretary of Health, Education and Welfare" and replaced it with "the President." [26]

On May 11, 1971, as the Senate Health Subcommittee prepared to mark up its final version of the cancer bill, the President issued a new statement on the cancer cure program. Noting again that "cancer has become one of mankind's deadliest and most elusive enemies," the President asked Congress to approve a specific cancer attack plan which differed "in a very important respect" from that under active consideration in the Senate. His proposal was for a program "within the National Institutes of Health and within the whole health establishment of the United States" but, simultaneously, a program "that is independently budgeted and is directly responsible to the President of the United States." He had chosen to take direct responsibility, the President explained, because of a deep personal interest in the cause and because of a conviction that "direct Presidential interest and Presidential guidance may hasten the day when we will find a cure for cancer." [27]

Very quickly, Senator Peter Dominick (R., Colo., after Javits the ranking Republican member of the Labor and Public Welfare Committee) introduced, on behalf of the Administration, S. 1828, spelling out details of the President's recommendation.[28] Almost as quickly, negotiations began between the Administration and the Senate sponsors of S. 34 to reconcile the differences between the two measures. Benno Schmidt, chairman of the original Senate panel of consultants, which had made the original proposition in November 1970, found himself representing the Senate as well as the panel—with the blessing of Senators Kennedy and Javits and Mrs. Lasker. Kenneth Cole was chief negotiator for the White House and the Administration. The Senate Health Subcommittee postponed final action on its original bill, which had been scheduled for the week the President made his decision. Subsequently, the committee scheduled hearings on the President's bill on June 8; and within two weeks S. 1828, as introduced by Senator Dominick on May 11, had been amended by striking out most of its original language and inserting the compromise language agreed upon by the Administration and the Committee. The Schmidt-Lasker bill had become in effect the Kennedy-Nixon bill, a most remarkable measure because of the unlikely alliance it seemed to symbolize. Another feature remarked upon by those who had watched the process carefully was that it seemed much more the cancer lobby's bill than the President's bill; further, "it was only through a last-minute maneuver that the Administration managed to retain some degree of influence—and political credit—in the Senate's decision on the structure of the program." [29]

While stating that the cancer cure program was to remain within the National Institutes of Health, in fact the "compromise measure," like the Kennedy-Javits bill, seemed to make it something apart: not only was its director to be a presidential appointee, approved by the Senate, and not only was he to control a budget which could be reviewed only at the level of the President, but he had no responsibility to report to or consult with the Director of NIH, and the Director effectively had nothing to say about the "Cancer Cure Program." The National Cancer Institute would be absorbed into the new cancer cure program. And as if to underscore the fact that the new effort was not merely an enlargement of the Cancer Institute's effort, an extensive search was immediately undertaken by the White House staff for a new director, with a principal criterion for selection being "managerial competence." [30] In short, even though the language of the compromise said the new program was to be part of NIH, it was given organizational and budgetary privileges tantamount to independence.

The full Senate Labor and Public Welfare Committee approved the "compromise" measure on June 16, and on July 7, over the protest of a lone Senator, Gaylord Nelson the Senate passed the bill by a vote of 79 to 1.

Dr. Merlin K. DuVal, Dean of the University of Arizona Medical School on leave to serve as Assistant Secretary of HEW for Health Affairs, remarked that Senator Nelson's vote was the loudest vote cast in the Senate in recent history.[31] Indeed, it seemed to become progressively louder as it echoed through the halls of academia and out to the people through editorials of some of the country's most important newspapers.

Still, the 79 aye votes seemed much louder, at that moment, than the one in opposition. And Senator Nelson's warning—that the separation of a new cancer research effort from the broader search for new knowledge and new cures might cause disintegration of the nation's splendid biomedical research enterprise and its primary government sponsor, NIH—seemed to strike little fear in most hearts, except the scientists'. The expectation was that, in 1971 as in 1937, the cancer bill at hand would go sailing through the House even faster than it had gone through the Senate.

The new cancer lobby, largely an extension of the old medical research lobby, seemed close to its greatest success. It had enlisted new friends including, and prominently so, the President of the United States, and even including some representatives of the new and potential rival lobby with its core of medical school and university faculties.

Some of the latter support had fallen away in the period since the effort had first begun. Dr. Joshua Lederberg, an original member of the Senate cancer panel, had written Senator Nelson before final Senate action to encourage Nelson in his opposition to the separation of cancer from other NIH efforts. Lederberg indicated that because he had agreed with the goals of the panel's report he had not at first objected to the means of achieving them; but on close re-examination he felt that even the elevation of cancer to a stronger budgetary position within NIH contained the seed of incipient disintegration of the NIH programs.[32]

Dr. Cooper of the medical colleges organization continued to press the theme he had adopted in the Senate hearings earlier that spring: "To proceed with the establishment of a cancer program separate from and independent of the essential process of scientific decision making represented by the National Institutes of Health would, we believe, gravely impair the objectives of a national attack upon cancer."[33]

Whether the establishment of an independent conquest of cancer agency, as proposed by the lobby spearheaded by Mary Lasker, would have changed the basic manner in which biomedical science is supported by the government and conducted by researchers is not provable. That it might lead to the disintegration of the NIH as we know it seemed quite plausible; the "heart people" were watching the congressional battle over cancer very closely, and were preparing to launch a campaign to elevate heart disease research—"after all heart disease kills more people than cancer"—if the cancer lobby was successful in their effort.[34] For NIH, the question was the same as it had been in 1945–46; the issue then as now was not whether the government would continue its support of biomedical research, but whether the NIH would be the agency given the primary job for coordinating that support. If the Conquest of Cancer Agency were established, a Conquest of Heart Disease Agency would be next, other separations would surely follow, and what was left of the National Institutes of Health would shrink into relative insignificance.

Organizational arrangements can affect policy outcomes, but the degree to which varying organizational forms affect the conduct of scientific research is not precisely measurable, especially if policy goals remain somewhat comprehensive and operational ethics remain constant. Thus it is conceivable that the establishment of a separate cancer authority would not radically have changed the nature of the American bioscientific enterprise, even though it probably would have changed dramatically the present government research support structure. Whether or not the new cancer research money was finally housed in a new independent agency or remained within NIH, certain traditions would have remained the same: although much of the money would be spent for contracts, many if not most such contracts would be with academic institutions; though a new emphasis was to be placed on targeted research, "targeted" research could encompass basic as well as applied research, for specific basic research gaps might be identified as needing targeted attention; and, in any case, basic research would receive a considerable portion of the additional money, which would principally be spent through the mechanism of academic research grants awarded only after peer review. The creation of an independent cancer research agency outside NIH might have made some marginal difference in the degree to which some researchers re-ordered the emphases of their work. But historical patterns suggest the probability that, even if some scientists followed the new cancer money to a new agency, most of them would change the titles of their proposed projects rather than the fundamental questions they wanted to investigate.

The old medical research lobby and its special cancer ex-tension—accustomed to the typical conservatism of the average scientist in forecasting practical health results from his care-fully delimited scientific research, and familiar with the medical research bureaucracy's tendency to initially oppose any big new governmental thrust—no doubt believed that once the new cancer agency was a political, scientific, and financial fact of life, the scientists and science administrators within and outside the federal government would adjust, and respond. Once more, historical patterns suggest that probability. But the cancer lobby failed to calculate the difference in size and so-phistication of the university-based science community in 1971 from that of the 1950's. The new sophistication included not only much wider awareness of how federal biomedical re-search policies are developed and how support programs are effectuated; it included as well a dramatic increase in willing-ness to try to affect such outcomes and not merely leave them to "political forces." Another important change had occurred since the medical research lobby began in the early fifties, with little help from the university community as a whole, to urge increased federal support for medical research through the National Institutes of Health: that agency had become the mother lode for the academic research community. As such, its immediate beneficiaries had become increasingly sensitive and responsive to the state of its political and fiscal health. "When NIH shivers," said Dr. Howard A. Schneider, of the University of North Carolina and the Federation of American Societies for Experimental Biology, to the Senate Health Subcommittee, "American biomedicine all over the country sneezes." [35]

When the Senate passed the Nixon-Kennedy bill in July, NIH shivered. And American biomedicine all over the country sneezed. With *Science* once more sounding the call, representatives of the institutions housing and the scientific societies representing American research scientists escalated their attack on the dismantling of NIH and the pseudo-scientists, lay meddlers, and misguided politicians leading the people down the primrose path of false hopes for a quick cure for cancer.

On the day the Senate passed the Nixon-Kennedy bill, Congressman Paul Rogers (D., Fla.) told his colleagues, in a speech on the floor of the House of Representatives, that he had serious doubts about the plan.[36] Rogers' reservations, like Senator Nelson's vote, became louder as they carried down the corridor of unfolding days. Rogers' position on the issue was important because his position in the House was important. With commencement of the Ninety-first Congress, he had become chairman of the Subcommittee on Public Health and Environment of the House Committee on Interstate and Foreign Commerce. A young man but a veteran of 16 years in Congress, Rogers had become particularly interested in the National Institutes of Health in 1965 when he had chaired a special subcommittee examining the organization of the Department of Health, Education and Welfare. His report to the committee and the House, filed in October 1966, contained a 25-page section on the NIH which was as balanced in its critique as it was short.[37] That report was overshadowed by the earlier and subsequent reports of the Fountain Committee, emphasizing NIH organizational weaknesses and management failures. But if it served no immediate practical purpose, the one-and-a-half-year study which preceded the report's issuance at least served to convince Rogers of the basic importance of the agency and the overall excellence of its programs. In classical form, a Congressman's particular assignment brought some specialized knowledge, which in turn led to keen personal interest.

Because of the open-ended appropriation enjoyed by NIH since 1944, the medical research lobby had not spent nearly as much time and effort becoming friends with the legislative committee members as with members of the appropriations committee. Rogers had never been sought out by Mrs. Lasker and her friends, principally because there had never been any need to seek his friendship. Thus his independent knowledge of the issue at hand was reinforced by his nonconnection with those who now sought what he believed was the first step in breaking up a first-class research agency. Further, he was surprised and annoyed and consequently even less susceptible to being caught up in the surging tide of political sentiment favoring a new cancer bureau, because in May he had introduced an identical bill to the Administration bill as introduced in the Senate by Senator Dominick, and then watched that proposal rapidly erode. Rogers served notice that he would not be stampeded and that his subcommittee would hold extensive hearings on the Senate-passed measure.

When the House committee hearings began in September, Mary Lasker was in the committee room. Concerned about Rogers' attitude, she went to see a friend whom she thought might be able to persuade him to relent: Congressman Harley Staggers (D., W. Va.), chairman of the full committee under whom Rogers served. There was no subsequent sign that Rogers' position had changed. The House hearings continued through the month and into October. Benno Schmidt and his panel colleagues having appeared immediately after the government witnesses, most of the fifty witnesses remaining were members of the biomedical science community. Their testimony was not only virtually unanimous, but adamant.[38] Rogers was clearly building a case against the Nixon-Kennedy-Schmidt-Lasker Bill and clearly waiting for popular passions to subside before he made his countermove. As if to undermine the position of his Senate counterpart, Rogers heard more testimony from scientists and doctors from Massachusetts than from any other single state.

Rogers and his subcommittee colleagues had other business in addition to the cancer matter. Also during the summer and fall of 1971, they forged and secured enactment of a major, straightforward federal program of support for medical education, a statute which had as its declared purpose the alleviation of physician shortages and shortages in related health professions, and which provided direct federal subsidies to institutions educating doctors, nurses, and related professionals.[39] In that matter as well as on the cancer bill, the House Health Subcommittee headed by Rogers found itself at odds with the Senate Health Subcommittee headed by Kennedy. A compromise on the issue was finally reached in October, after several meetings of the House and Senate conferees; the final product seemed closer to the House version than to that adopted by the Senate.

The House committee was also working on legislation, keenly desired by the Administration, to set up a special White House Action Office for Drug Abuse Prevention, thus attesting presidential interest and leadership in another area of national concern. It seemed possible, as the fall unfolded, that there might be no cancer bill enacted in 1971 despite presidential dramatization of the issue, popular interest in it, Senate action on it, and the urgent desire of the cancer lobby to achieve the final organizational victory which they had intermittently sought and which had previously eluded them but which now seemed so close at hand. At the suggestion of the honorary chairman of the

American Cancer Society, Mary Lasker, the Society raised funds for full-page ads in major newspapers across the country and in some less-than-major newspapers located in the congressional districts of the Rogers subcommittee members.[40] The Message addressed to the people implied that a small handful of willful men in the House were hamstringing the effort, staunchly supported by the President and the Senate, to conquer cancer. If the advertisement created greater awareness of the issue among the people, it created sharp indignation among the members of the House subcommittee. Rogers and other House members suggested that the American Cancer Society might have jeopardized its right to tax-exempt status by spending such large sums in such a blatant attempt to influence votes.[41] The President of the Cancer Society apologized to the House members thus offended, and various friends and colleagues of Mrs. Lasker whispered that they had tried mightily to talk her out of running the ad in the first place.

Other approaches were tried. Colonel Luke Quinn, veteran lobbyist of the Cancer Society, called all his old House friends from his hospital bed, where he was confined for treatment of cancer. Mike Gorman searched for soft spots in the health subcommittee and in the full committee, proposing various ways that House members could move closer to the Senate bill without losing face. For once, he met total resistance. Legislative liaison specialists from the HEW and the White House separately conferred with subcommittee chairman Rogers and his staff, similarly suggesting possible openings, and similarly failing. Secretary Richardson wrote to Congressman Staggers saying that the Administration now was fully behind the measure passed by the Senate and urging House adoption of it,[42] a move he was shortly to regret, for the Administration in fact adopted two more positions on the issue before the final agreement was reached.

The principal effect of the cancer lobby's last round of efforts to influence votes in the House seemed to be the opposite of that desired: the health subcommittee position solidified in its opposition to any proposal which would remove the new cancer attack from the National Cancer Institute. Ironically, that position was basically the one proposed by the President in May, and one which the Administration now tried to undermine: The House committee rejected creation of a new cancer bureau incorporating the existing Cancer Institute, with a new super-grade director. Instead, the House insisted that the expanded cancer effort be carried on within the NCI. As the Nixon-Dominick bill had proposed, the Rogers bill permitted the Cancer Institute to have an independent budget, to be changed only at the presidential level but requiring that the Director of the National Institutes of Health and the Secretary of HEW comment upon it. That still meant considerable independence for the cancer program, and it answered the argument of the cancer lobby that the levels of bureaucracy and budget review retard the victory against the disease.

Some thought that there was little difference in the effects on NIH of the House formulation and the potential effects of the Senate formulation, for cancer was clearly to have a "most-favored program" status in either case. Removing control of the cancer budget from NIH was to remove the most effective control, notwithstanding the fact that the Director of the Cancer Institute otherwise reported to the NIH Director. Still, no new bureau, agency, or institute was to be created; no new generalissimos were to be given new commands. Besides, most scientists and their representatives felt the House proposal was a better arrangement, and the medical science bureaucracy knew it was the best deal they could get, given existing political circumstances.

Having denied the President a cancer attack director reporting directly to him, as the Senate Bill would have provided, the House committee did include in their final draft a provision for a three-man "Cancer Attack Panel," to be appointed by the President and that would keep him regularly and directly informed of progress, problems, and needs. This item, proposed by Congressman Ancher Nelson of Minnesota, ranking minority member of the subcommittee, firmed up his endorsement of the bill, and it was reported by unanimous vote to the full committee. With the norm of subcommittee unity based on prior bipartisan agreement thus firmly in place, the brief urgings of two fellow members of the full committee made no impact, and the bill was approved by the Interstate and Foreign Committee by a vote of 26 to 2. Chairman Harley Staggers himself reported that vote to the House in urging adoption of the bill he had himself not favored.[43]

When the bill came to the floor of the House, John Rooney, one of John Fogarty's old Irish brigade, Robert Tiernan, who succeeded Fogarty as congressman from the First Congressional District of Rhode Island, and Brock Adams (D., Wash.) were among a few who sought in vain to persuade their colleagues that more dramatic changes in the existing machinery were needed to produce scientific breakthroughs in cancer. Tiernan urged the House to support the President, rather than the House Commerce Committee. But the ranking Republican of that committee, William Springer of Illinois, replied that the gentleman from Rhode Island was mistaken, for the President supported the bill reported by the House committee.

> Congressman Tiernan: Is it not true that the President approved the Senate bill as passed?
> Congressman Springer: He approves this bill.
> Tiernan: But the President also approves the Senate bill.
> Springer: I said the President approves this bill.

Jake Pickle, Lyndon Johnson's congressman who also supported the Schmidt-Lasker-Nixon-Kennedy bill, sought to clarify the issue:

> Congressman Pickle: Mr. Speaker, my question is: Does the President prefer this bill or does he accept it?

Congressman Springer: All he said was that it is a good bill, and he approves it.

Pickle: I think there is a great deal of difference.[44]

If the call to rally around "the President's position" evoked no support in the House, it may have been because the President's exact position was difficult to ascertain. As Congressman Staggers recalled: "The Administration appears to have taken four different positions. At first they were opposed to any legislation; then they proposed their own bill; they appeared before our committee and supported the Senate bill; and the last of their positions is support of the Senate bill with a substantial number of amendments adopted by the Subcommittee on Public Health and the Environment" (p. 11012).

Congressman James Hastings (R., N.Y.), a member of the health subcommittee who had been particularly active in assisting Rogers to steer the bill to passage, volunteered an explanation: "The President, unfortunately, in consideration of the Senate bill did not have the advantage of knowing that the House would come up with this superior piece of legislation" (p. 11018).

There was, in the end, no fight. Congressman Claude Pepper, Mary Lasker's longtime ally and Congress' most persistent advocate of new governmental initiatives against cancer, merely expressed the hope that a conference committee would work out a final measure which contained some of the Senate's suggestions. In that vain hope, he voted for the House measure. The final vote was 350 to 5 (pp. 11018–11019, 11026).

The cancer lobby had had its day in the Senate. Those claiming to represent American biomedical science had had their day in the House. Paul Rogers reported to his colleagues, before the final vote, on who was behind the bill he had shepherded through his subcommittee, the full committee, and onto the floor of the House:

The president of the National Academy of Sciences, as well as the Academy of Medicine of the National Academy of Sciences, have stated strong support of this approach. Scores of national organizations, including the American Medical Association, the American Hospital Association, and the Association of American Medical Colleges, as well as practically every significant scientific body in the United States, supported the concept of maintaining the Federal cancer research effort within the NIH. Several recipients of the Nobel prize in medicine, including a Nobel laureate whose award was based on his treatment of cancer patients, expressed support of the approach contained in this bill. Heads of 72 medicine departments of medical schools throughout the country expressed approval of the committee's approach. Thirteen faculty members of Harvard Medical School, each long associated in cancer research, or treatment of cancer patients, publicly supported the course of action contemplated in this bill (p. 11013).

With that combination arrayed against the Nixon-Kennedy bill, it is not surprising that the conference committee ultimately agreed upon a bill which, despite the similar purpose of the originals, looked more like the House measure than like that passed by the Senate with the President's specific blessing. Not that the new medical research lobby simply represented a larger constituency—the biomedical researchers—than the old medical research lobby with Mrs. Lasker and her friends at its center. Indeed, the cancer group within that larger lobby, especially including the American Cancer Society, claimed to represent millions of actual and potential victims of the disease. Nor was the new lobby's success related to its greater energy or more ingenious strategy. The core reason was that, for the first time in several decades of lobbying for more funds or new directions in federal support of medical research, the scientists themselves joined issue with their would-be benefactors and opposed them.

That the proposal for a new cancer research agency with some degree of autonomy got as far as it did in the policy process in 1971 reflects the fact that it had some support in the scientific community. As Congressman Staggers reported: "it would appear that the majority of cancer researchers advocated the approach of the Senate bill." But the reason that approach did not make it all the way through the policy process was that, "virtually to a man, the remainder of the scientific community is opposed to the separation of the cancer program from NIH, and favors the approach contained in H. R. 11302, the final House measure" (p. 11012).

When the conference between the House committee and the Senate committee got under way, the principal spokesmen for the Senate, Senators Kennedy and Javits, tried to retain as many of their bill's provisions as possible. But messages had already been transmitted that some of the Senate conferees now favored the House position. To the chagrin of Ted Kennedy, Gaylord Nelson openly urged his House counterparts not to concede certain points under discussion, saying they would win the points if they stuck to their guns.[45]

Nor did the President bolster the Senate conferees' hand. Asked by Harrison Williams (D., N.J.), chairman of the full Senate committee, to state his position one more time, the President wrote to Williams as the conference committee began, saying that he saw merit in both measures and that what he wanted most of all was some bill to sign so that the new attack on cancer could be launched. Their positions thus weakened by the President's refusal to state further preferences—and weakened from within by new doubts occasioned by the strong opposition of much of the medical science community to their earlier action—the Senate conferees conceded on most points of difference, and Congress finally enacted, on November 15, the Cancer Act of 1971.[46]

The 1971 Cancer Act—"a Christmas present for the American

people," said Congressman Rogers[47]—authorized the government to spend $1.59 billion in cancer research over a three-year period. It elevated the National Advisory Cancer Council to a National Cancer Board comprised of five federal government officials (including the Secretary of HEW and the Director of NIH) and 19 members appointed by the President. The Senate had followed Mrs. Lasker's preference that half the members be laymen; but the House prevailed, so that only one-third of the presidential appointees are not scientists or physicians, as is currently the case with the other advisory councils. The Director of the National Cancer Institute (and the Director of the National Institutes of Health) will henceforth be appointed by the President, rather than the NIH Director being appointed by the Secretary of HEW and the Cancer Institute Director named by the NIH Director. The three-man Cancer Attack Panel authorized must include "one panelist skilled in management" and two distinguished scientists or physicians.[48]

The President launched the newest crusade against cancer on the day before Christmas Eve. Cautioning that "biomedical research is, of course, a notoriously uncertain enterprise," President Nixon nonetheless expressed belief that progress would now be made, both because of recent scientific advances and because the new Act permitted the President "to take personal command of the federal effort to conquer cancer so that its activities need not be stymied by the familiar dangers of bureaucracy and red tape."[49] The emergent new congressional health leaders, Paul Rogers and Ted Kennedy, were present at the signing, as were members of Senator Yarborough's cancer panel of 1970, officials of the American Cancer Society, and the directors of the National Institutes of Health. Mary Lasker looked on, beaming.

Dr. Clarence C. Little, director of research of the American Society for the Control of Cancer, whom Mrs. Lasker had thought was too conservative in 1942, died of a heart attack the day before the President signed the Cancer Act at age 83.[50]

Dr. Rolla E. Dyer, Director of the National Institutes of Health in the 1940's, who the emerging medical research lobby thought was retarding progress against dread disease in that era, had died six months earlier, aged 84.[51] Their positions on the new crusade are not recorded. But if Matthew Neely could have heard the President's words, he surely would have applauded from the grave: "As this year comes to an end, cancer remains one of mankind's deadliest and most elusive enemies. Each year it takes more lives in this country alone than we lost in battle in all of World War II. Its long shadow of fear darkens every corner of the earth. But just as cancer represents a grim threat to men and women and children in all parts of the world, so the launching of our great crusade against cancer should be the cause of new hope among people everywhere." [52]

The legislative act and the presidential pronouncement signaled more than the launching of the crusade, however. For one thing, the Act restored the right of the legislative committees of Congress to make periodic authorizations for cancer research, a perogative they had lost to the appropriations committees in 1948 and which the appropriations committees had no interest in losing back to them. For another, the President named as chairman of the Cancer Attack Panel, Benno Schmidt, the Johnny-come-lately who had raised the hackles of NIH officials in his complaints about the bureaucracy and whose friendship with Mary Lasker guaranteed that zealous first member of the Crusade an important access which some of her critics hoped and thought she had surely lost for good.

The President broadly acknowledged "the hard and careful effort which so many members of Congress gave to this cause" and expressed pleasure that the program they had enacted "incorporates the basic recommendations I made last May." [53] But singled out for special praise was the American Cancer Society, which organization had placed an ad attacking Congressman Rogers' position on the cancer issue in his hometown newspaper just a few months earlier. The President's sobriquet to the

Cancer Society could not have pleased the Congressman. Nor could the key Senators have been pleased that some commentators were already referring to the new statute as primarily the work of Congressman Rogers and were suggesting that Rogers had won the right to wear the health leadership mantle of John Fogarty and Lister Hill.

If some differences had been reconciled and a common goal agreed upon in the Cancer Act of 1971, it seemed certain that several old struggles were about to begin anew: struggles between a reinvigorated medical research lobby and a newly assertive biomedical science community; between those who now had new justification for concentrating only on one specific policy goal and those who would automatically interpret the mandate broadly; between the elected public official and the science research bureaucrat; between rival political figures, opposing political parties, and jealously co-equal branches of the national government. Simultaneously, the struggle was renewed between all those men and institutions and cancer itself, that dread disease, insatiable monster, implacable foe.

Notes   Index

Notes

Chapter I. Conquering Cancer: The Origins of a National Policy

1. U.S., Congress, Senate, *Congressional Record,* 70th Cong., 1st sess., 1928, 69, pt. 8:9048.
2. *Ibid.*
3. *Ibid.,* pp. 9049–9050.
4. *Ibid.,* p. 950.
5. *Ibid.*
6. T. Harry Williams, *Huey Long* (New York: Alfred A. Knopf, 1969), p. 219.
7. Donald C. Swain, "The Rise of a Research Empire," *Science,* 14 Dec. 1962, p. 1233.
8. Ora Marashino, comp., "National Cancer Institute Historical Materials," 1:1–3, National Cancer Institute History Division, Bethesda, Md.
9. *Congressional Record,* 70th Cong., 1st sess., 1928, 69, pt. 8:9050.
10. *Ibid.,* p. 9049. It is surprising that no one among the 11 doctors and professors who helped Senator Neely formulate his 1928 plan thought enough—if they knew—of the PHS efforts to propose that agency's inclusion in the study. The 11 included, among others: Drs. J. B. Murphy of the Rockefeller Institute, Lewis H. Weed, Roland Park, and Bloodgood of Johns Hopkins.
11. *Ibid.,* p. 9050.
12. Richard H. Shyrock, *American Medical Research* (New York: Commonwealth Fund, 1947), p. 44.
13. Daniel S. Greenberg, *The Politics of Pure Science* (New York: New American Library, 1967), p. 44.
14. Bess Furman, "A Profile of the Public Health Service of the United States," unpub. ms., National Library of Medicine, History of Medicine Division, 1969, chap. x, p. 29.
15. *Ibid.,* chap. xi, p. 11.
16. Shyrock, *American Medical Research,* p. 101. Shyrock attempted to ascertain how much of the $12.2 million spent for medicine and public health by all private foundations in 1940 went for research but was apparently unable to do so. He doubted the validity of the estimate suggested by the Wartime Subcommittee on Health (offered in 1944) of $5 million from both public and private funds, believing that figure too low.
17. *Congressional Record,* 70th Cong., 1st sess., 1928, 69, pt. 8:9050.
18. Marashino, "NCI Historical Materials," 1:1–3.
19. Neely ran again for the Senate in 1930 and was re-elected. He served until 1941, when he resigned to assume the governorship to which he was elected while still in the Senate. Thereafter he served again in the Senate (1948–1954), and in the House (1945–1947) just after completing his

term as Governor of West Virginia. He continued to push cancer research with mixed success.

20. *Ibid.,* pp. 8–10.

21. *Ibid.,* pp. 12–13.

22. *Congressional Record,* 70th Cong., 1st sess., 1928, 69, pt. 8:9051.

23. *Ibid.*

24. 46 *Stat.* 379 (Public Law 71-251).

25. See Marashino, "NCI Historical Materials" generally; Furman, "Profile of the Public Health Service," chap. xvi, pp. 11–12. See also memorandum of Assistant Surgeon General L. R. Thompson, 26 May 1938, written for the cornerstone of the new NIH building, in files of the Historian of NIH (Dr. Winn Miles), Bethesda, Md.

26. Swain, "The Rise of a Research Empire," p. 1234.

27. *Ibid.*

28. Furman, "Profile of the Public Health Service," chap. xvi, p. 7.

29. L. R. Thompson, memorandum for NIH building cornerstone.

30. Swain, "The Rise of a Research Empire," p. 1234.

31. Marashino, "NCI Historical Materials," 2:6.

32. *Ibid.,* p. 10.

33. *Ibid.,* pp. 12–17 *passim.*

34. Letter from Saul Haas to Dr. J. R. Heller, Director of the National Cancer Institute, 1 March 1955, NCI History Division.

35. Marashino, "NCI Historical Materials," 2:25–28.

36. *Ibid.,* p. 30.

37. *Ibid.,* p. 30.

38. U.S. Congress, Committees on Commerce of the Senate and House, *Joint Hearings on Cancer Research,* 75th Cong., 1st sess., 8 July 1937, pp. 28, 50–51.

39. Marashino, "NCI Historical Materials," 2:25–28.

40. *Ibid.,* p. 30.

41. 50 *Stat.* 559 (P.L. 75-244).

42. *Joint Hearings on Cancer Research,* 75th Cong., 1st sess., 8 July 1937, pp. 63–71.

43. *Journal of the American Medical Association,* 109, no. 16, 16 Oct. 1937.

44. Haas letter to Heller.

45. Oscar Ewing, Federal Security Administrator, to Senator Royal Copeland, chairman of the Senate Commerce Committee, 3 July 1937, quoted in Marashino, "NCI Historical Materials," 2:39.

Chapter II. The War Years and Reconversion: Hazards and Possibilities

1. Under the new arrangement, Dr. James R. Conant became chairman of the Weapons Committee, with Bush heading the Office of Scientific Research and Development. Chester S. Keefer, "Dr. Richards as Chairman of the Committee on Medical Research," *Annals of Internal Medicine,* vol. 71, no. 5, pt. 2, November 1969. See also Irwin Stewart, *Organizing Scientific Research for War* (Boston: Little, Brown, 1948); and U.S. Congress, Senate, Committee on Education and Labor, *Hearings on Wartime Health and Education,* 78th Cong., 2nd sess., 2 Jan. 1945, pp. 2196–2198.

2. Keefer, "Dr. Richards and CMR," pp. 61–70 *passim*.

3. *Ibid.*, p. 62.

4. *Ibid.*, pp. 62–63.

5. A. N. Richards, quoted in Keefer, "Dr. Richards and CMR," p. 61.

6. U.S., Congress, Senate, Committee on Education and Labor, *Report on Wartime Health and Education*, report no. 3, 78th Cong., 2nd sess., 2 Jan. 1945, p. 20.

7. *Hearings on Wartime Health and Education*, 78th Cong., 2nd sess., p. 2198.

8. *Ibid.*, p. 2208.

9. Keefer, "Dr. Richards and CMR," p. 69.

10. Vannevar Bush, *Science: The Endless Frontier* (Washington: U.S. Office of Scientific Research and Development, 1945; rep., National Science Foundation, July 1960), p. 3.

11. U.S. Congress, P.L. 410, 78th Cong., 2nd sess., 1944.

12. *Hearings on Wartime Health and Education*, 78th Cong., 2nd sess. (testimony of Gen. Lewis Hershey), 10 July 1944, p. 1620.

13. *Ibid.*, 15 Dec. 1944, p. 2240.

14. Donald C. Swain, "The Rise of a Research Empire," *Science*, 14 Dec. 1962, p. 1233.

15. *Hearings on Wartime Health and Education*, p. 2276.

16. *Report on Wartime Health and Education*, report no. 3, p. 20.

17. President Truman's objections caused him to veto the first version of the National Science Foundation in 1947.

18. *Journal of the American Medical Association*, 3 Nov. 1945, p. 699.

19. Swain, "Rise of a Research Empire," p. 1237.

20. *Public Papers of the Presidents of the U.S.: Harry S Truman* (12 April to 31 Dec. 1945): "Special Message Presenting a 21-Point Program for the Reconversion Period" (no. 128), 6 Sept. 1945 (Washington: Government Printing Office, 1961), p. 203.

21. *Ibid.*, p. 294.

22. *Public Papers of the Presidents: Harry S Truman*: "Special Message to the Congress Recommending a Comprehensive Health Program" (no. 192), 19 Nov. 1945, pp. 514–515.

23. U.S. Congress, Senate, Committee on Military Affairs, *Hearings on Science Legislation*, 78th Cong., 1st sess., 23 Oct. 1945, pp. 514–515.

24. Swain, "Rise of a Research Empire," p. 1235: Dyer to Richards, 29 Aug. 1944, National Archives, Records of the Committee on Medical Research, Demobilization File.

25. Swain, "Rise of a Research Empire"; Dyer letter to Richards.

26. E.g., Ronald C. Moe and Steven C. Teel, "Congress as Policy-Maker: A Necessary Reappraisal," *Political Science Quarterly*, 75 (September 1970), 443–470.

27. Daniel S. Greenberg, *The Politics of Pure Science* (New York: New American Library, 1967), p. 104. It is probable though not absolutely certain that Dr. Bush drafted the letter from President Roosevelt to himself, asking for a plan for postwar support of science. Dr. Bush himself does not remember firmly whether he did so. He recently wrote: "I suppose I wrote the letter; that was common procedure" (Bush to Strickland, 10 Nov. 1970). For a description of the Kilgore proposal, see J. L. Penick, Jr., C. W. Pursell, Jr., M. B. Sherwood, and D. C. Swain, eds., *The Politics of*

American Science: 1930 to Present (Chicago: Rand McNally, 1965), pp. 34–47 *passim.*

28. Memorandum from Dr. R. E. Dyer, acting director of Hygienic Laboratory, to Surgeon General Hugh S. Cumming, 28 Aug. 1926, p. 3, files of the NIH Historian, Bethesda, Md.

29. Memorandum from Dr. Stimson to Dr. Cumming, 23 March 1929, files of the NIH Historian.

30. Memorandum from Dr. McCoy to Dr. Cumming, undated, files of the NIH Historian.

31. Dyer memo, p. 1.

32. Victor H. Kramer, "The National Institutes of Health: A Study in Administration" (1937), files of the NIH Historian.

33. Swain, "Rise of a Research Empire," p. 1234.

34. *Hearings on Wartime Health and Education,* 78th Cong., 1st sess., 14 Dec. 1944, p. 2177.

35. Bush, *Science: The Endless Frontier,* p. 16.

36. John R. Steelman, *Science and Public Policy: A Program for the Nation,* Report to the President, 17 Oct. 1947, V, 113.

37. 46 *Stat.* 379 (P.L. 71-251).

38. Dyer to Richards, 29 Aug. 1944, National Archives, OSRD Demobilization File.

39. Figures for NIH budgets are found in many sources. For simplicity and consistency, unless otherwise indicated, I have used those figures contained in the *NIH Almanac, 1969* (Bethesda, Md.: NIH Office of Information), Appropriations Table, p. 81.

40. Kenneth M. Endicott and Ernest M. Allen, "The Growth of Medical Research, 1941–1953, and the Role of Public Health Service Grants," *Science,* 25 Sept. 1953, p. 341.

Chapter III. The Rise of the Research Lobby: A New Mobilization

1. Descriptions of Mr. and Mrs. Lasker's and Mrs. Mahoney's involvement in the medical research effort, contained in this chapter, are based on a number of sources, including numerous interviews over the past five years with the two women and with other key figures such as former Surgeon General Leonard Scheele and U.S. Congressman (earlier Senator) Claude Pepper. The Laskers' interest in medical research and some of their early activities have been detailed in John Gunther's biography of Albert Lasker, *Taken at the Flood* (New York: Harper, 1960), upon which I have relied for some purposes. For points of central importance, I have attempted to secure corroboration of accuracy from more than one source. "Statements of fact" contained in this chapter which are not specifically attributed to a single source are based on cumulative evidence developed in the course of several years' research.

2. For example, from inception of the Albert Lasker Awards for basic and clinical research in 1946 (first through the American Public Health Association and for the past decade directly through the Lasker Foundation), 22 Lasker award winners had become Nobel Prize winners by 1972.

3. Albert Lasker's life, like Mary's, was one into which illness constantly intruded. His first wife was ill off and on from the time they married in

1902 to the time she died in 1936. Lasker died of cancer in 1952, leaving half of his $11-million estate to his widow and half to the Albert and Mary Lasker Foundation.

4. Quoted in Daniel S. Greenberg, *The Politics of Pure Science* (New York: The New American Library, 1967), p. 134.

5. *Ibid.*

6. Richard H. Shyrock, *American Medical Research* (New York: The Commonwealth Fund, 1947), p. 104.

7. *Ibid.*

8. U.S., Congress, Senate, Committee on Education and Labor, *Hearing on Wartime Health and Education*, 78th Cong., 1st sess. (December 1944), p. iii (hereafter cited as *Pepper committee hearings*).

9. *Ibid.*, p. 2241.

10. *Ibid.*, pp. 2275–2276.

11. John Gunther, a longtime friend of the Laskers, states in his biography of Albert (p. 318) that it was Mary's memo to Anna Rosenberg, which Mrs. Rosenberg passed along to the President, that prompted FDR to "turn the matter over to Judge Rosenman, who promptly wrote a letter in FDR's name to Dr. Bush, directing him to prepare a report." Dan Greenberg suggests that Dr. Bush initiated the presidential request—in no small part because he was concerned about an idea of Senator Harley Kilgore (D., W. Va.) for government support for science after the war. Bush thought Kilgore's draft plan would too heavily involve political judgments and would set up "a gadgeteer's paradise." Greenberg, *Politics of Pure Science*, p. 105n. In a letter dated 10 Nov. 1970, Dr. Bush comments on the matter: "There was never any question about the inclusion of medical research when my report to FDR was being prepared. Medical research was a part of OSRD, and none needed to suggest it be included."

12. Vannevar Bush, *Science: The Endless Frontier* (Washington: U.S. Office of Scientific Research and Development, 1945; rep., National Science Foundation, 1960), p. 3.

13. Truman vetoed the bill, introduced by Senator Magnuson and supported by most scientists, that was enacted in 1947; the President believed it provided inadequate government control over federal support for science.

14. Dr. Dyer was perceived by some members of the House Appropriations Subcommittee handling NIH appropriations to be just the opposite of the conservative, overly cautious scientist. In the fiscal 1947 appropriations hearings, Dyer boldly asked the committee to provide an extra $3 million which the Budget Bureau had not approved. Queried as to whether he would accept less than that, Dyer said he must have it all or postpone critically important research. "I do not myself feel justified in taking the responsibility for postponing anything in the matter of medical research," he told the committee. "If Sir Alexander Fleming had delayed 1 year in starting his research on penicillin, you can add up for yourselves the number of lives that would have been lost." Labor FSA Appropriations Hearings, 1947, House, 79th Cong., 2nd sess., p. 180. Perhaps Dyer had detected the strength and direction of the political winds by the time of these hearings.

15. U.S., Congress, House, H.R. 4502, 79th Cong., 2nd sess.

16. *Pepper committee hearings*, pp. 2200–2201.

17. *Ibid.*, p. 2259.

18. Interview with Dr. Scheele, 12 Feb. 1970.

19. 60 *Stat.* 421 (P.L. 79-487).

20. Transcript of oral interview with Dr. Robert Felix by Harlan Phillips, February 1963 (National Library of Medicine, History of Medicine Division), esp. pp. 39–40. See also Jeanne L. Brand, "The National Mental Health Act of 1946: A Retrospect," *Bulletin of the History of Medicine,* vol. 39 (May–June 1965). Dr. Felix recalls having to obtain a grant from the Greentree Foundation to pay expenses for the first meeting of the Mental Health Advisory Council.

21. Bess Furman, "A Profile of the Public Health Service of the United States," unpub. ms., National Library of Medicine, History of Medicine Division, 1969, chap. xvii, p. 33.

22. U.S., Congress, House, Committee on Appropriations, *Hearings on Labor-Federal Security Agency Appropriations, 1947,* 79th Cong., 2nd sess., pp. 290–291.

23. Interview with Dr. Scheele.

24. *Labor-FSA Hearings, 1947,* p. 291.

25. U.S., Congress, House, Committee on Foreign Affairs, *Hearings on Mobilization of World's Cancer Experts,* 79th Cong., 2nd sess., May 1946, pp. 5–6.

26. Interviews with Dr. Scheele, Congressman Pepper, et al.

27. *Science and Public Policy: A Program for the Future,* Report of the President's Scientific Research Board (Steelmen Report), 17 Oct. 1945, V, 9.

28. Furman, "Profile of PHS," chap. xix, pp. 12–13.

29. Greenberg, *Politics of Pure Science,* p. 200.

30. 62 *Stat.* 464 (P.L. 80-635).

Chapter IV. Federal Aid for Medical Education: The AMA and Avenues Blocked

1. Richard Harris, *A Sacred Trust* (New York: New American Library, 1966). See also Stanley Kelley, Jr., *Professional Public Relations and Political Power* (Baltimore: Johns Hopkins Press, 1965), esp. chap. iii; Herman R. Somers and Anne R. Somers, *Doctors, Patients, and Health Insurance* (Washington: Brookings Institution, 1961); Elton Ryack, *Professional Power and American Medicine* (Baltimore: Johns Hopkins Press, 1963). For treatments of the AMA as a political interest group generally, see Oliver Garceau, *The Political Life of the American Medical Association* (Hamden, Conn.: Archon Books, 1961); and David B. Truman, *The Governmental Process: Political Interests and Public Opinion* (New York: Alfred A. Knopf, 1967), esp. pp. 170–171.

2. *Public Papers of the Presidents of the United States: Harry S Truman:* "Special Message to the Congress Recommending a Comprehensive Health Program" (no. 128), 19 Nov. 1945 (Washington: Government Printing Office, 1961).

3. U.S., Congress, Senate, *Congressional Record,* 82nd Cong., 1st sess., 1951 (Albert Q. Maisel, "Our Alarming Doctor Shortage"), 97, pt. 10: 12526.

4. *Ibid.*

5. U.S., Congress, House, Committee on Interstate and Foreign Commerce, *Hearings on National Health Plan,* 81st Cong., 1st sess., 24 May 1949, p. 50 (cited hereafter as *House Hearings on National Health Plan*).

6. U.S., Congress, Senate, Committee on Labor and Public Welfare, *Hearings on National Health Program, 1949,* 81st Cong., 1st sess., p. 639 (cited hereafter as *Senate Hearings on National Health Program*).

7. *Ibid.,* pp. 209, 210–211.

8. *Ibid.,* p. 116.

9. *Ibid.,* pp. 28ff.

10. *Ibid.,* p. 30.

11. *Ibid.,* p. 217.

12. *Ibid.,* p. 208.

13. *Ibid.,* p. 211.

14. *Ibid.,* p. 205.

15. *Ibid.*

16. *Congressional Record,* 82nd Cong., 1st sess., 1951 (Maisel article) 97, pt. 10:12527.

17. *Senate Hearings on National Health Program,* p. 117.

18. *Congressional Record,* 81st Cong., 1st sess., 1949, 95, pt. 10:13225.

19. *Ibid.,* p. 13229.

20. *Congressional Record,* 82nd Cong., 1st sess., 1951, 97, pt. 10:12527.

21. *Ibid.*

22. *Ibid.*

23. *Ibid.*

24. *Ibid.*

25. *Ibid.,* p. 12528.

26. *Ibid.*

27. *Medical School Grants and Finances,* Report of the Surgeon General's Committee on Medical School Grants and Finances (Washington: Government Printing Office, 1951), pt. 1:46.

28. *Congressional Record,* 82nd Cong., 1st sess., 1951, 97, pt. 10:12514.

29. *Ibid.,* p. 12576.

30. *Ibid.,* p. 2236.

31. *Ibid.,* pt. 10:12514.

32. *Ibid.,* pt. 2:2237.

33. *Ibid.*

34. *Ibid.,* pt. 10:12514.

35. *Ibid.,* p. 12545.

36. *Ibid.,* p. 12547.

37. *Ibid.,* p. 12545.

38. *Ibid.,* p. 12547.

39. *Ibid.,* p. 12581.

40. *Ibid.*

41. *Ibid.,* p. 12582.

42. *Ibid.*

43. There was no southern bloc in action here, however. Some southern Senators favored the Kerr-Russell amendment and some didn't; and southerners were similarly divided on the bill itself.

44. *Congressional Record,* 82nd Cong., 1st sess., 1951, 97, pt. 10:12581.

45. *Ibid.,* p. 22579.

46. *Ibid.*, p. 12579.

47. *Journal of the American Medical Association,* 15 Dec. 1951, p. 1576. The quotations that follow are from pp. 1576, 1577, 1579.

Chapter V. Emerging Congressional Leadership

1. On source of figures for NIH appropriations, see above, Chapter II, n. 39.

2. Stephen P. Strickland, "The Origins and Consequences of Subcommittee Unity: An Analysis of Labor-HEW Appropriations Bills, 1954–66," unpub. diss., Johns Hopkins University, 1966.

3. U.S., Congress, House, Committee on Appropriations, *Hearings on Labor-Federal Security Appropriations, 1947,* 79th Cong., 2nd sess., "Public Health Service," p. 187 (cited hereafter as *House Appropriations Hearings*).

4. Public Health Service Act of 1944, 58 *Stat.* 682 (P.L. 78-410).

5. Interview with Dr. Leonard Scheele, 12 Feb. 1970.

6. *Ibid.*

7. Richard Fenno, *The Power of the Purse: Appropriations Politics in Congress* (Boston: Little, Brown, 1966), esp. chaps. i and ii.

8. *House Appropriations Hearings, 1950,* 81st Cong., 1st sess., "Public Health Service," January 1949.

9. U.S., Congress, House, *Congressional Record,* 81st Cong., 2nd sess., 1950, 96, pt. 5:5843.

10. *House Appropriations Hearings, 1950,* 81st Cong., 1st sess., "Public Health Service," p. 303.

11. *Ibid.*, p. 347. The quotations that follow are from pp. 348, 349, 352.

12. U.S., Congress, House, Committee on Appropriations, *Report on Labor-FSA Appropriations, 1950,* 81st Cong., 1st sess.

13. *Congressional Record,* 81st Cong., 1st sess., 1949, 95, pt. 4:5122.

14. Omnibus Medical Research Act of 1950, 64 *Stat.* 443 (P.L. 81-692).

15. Alan T. Waterman, to new edition of *Science: The Endless Frontier* (Washington: National Science Foundation, 1960), p. xii.

16. *Ibid.*, p. xi.

17. *House Appropriations Hearings, 1951,* 81st Cong., 2nd sess., "Public Health Service," p. 129. Note: The Department of Health, Education and Welfare was created in 1953 and absorbed the Federal Security Agency; hence designation of the hearings as "Labor-HEW Appropriations" beginning with fiscal 1954.

18. Waterman, *Science: The Endless Frontier,* p. xii.

19. A quick summary of Fenno's concept can be gained by reading *Power of the Purse,* pp. 262–263, 500–501. A detailed analysis of the practical political reasons prompting compliance with the "norm of subcommittee unity" is provided in Strickland, "The Origins and Consequences of Subcommittee Unity."

20. *House Appropriations Hearings, 1951,* 81st Cong., 2nd sess., "Public Health Service," p. 518.

21. *Ibid.*

22. *Congressional Record,* 81st Cong., 1st sess., 1950, 96, pt. 5:5801.

23. *Ibid.*, 83rd Cong., 2nd sess., 1954, 100, pt. 6:7856.
24. *Ibid.*, p. 7869.
25. *Ibid.*, p. 8006.
26. *Ibid.*, 1st sess., 1953, pt. 6:8060.
27. U.S., Congress, Senate, Committee on Appropriations, *Hearings on Labor-HEW Appropriations, 1961*, 86th Cong., 1st sess., "Public Health Service," p. 1429 (cited hereafter as *Senate Appropriations Hearings*).
28. *Brown v. Board of Education*, 34 U.S. 483, 98 L. Ed. 873 (1954).
29. Transcript of oral interview with Senator Hill by Harlan Phillips, National Library of Medicine, History of Medicine Division, 1967, p. 21.
30. *New York Times*, 28 Jan. 1968, p. 28.
31. Interview with Sen. Hruska, 23 Aug. 1965.
32. According to Senator Hill and others. See Stephen Horn, *Unused Power: The Work of the Senate Committee on Appropriations* (Washington: Brookings Institution, 1970).
33. *Congressional Record*, 81st Cong., 1st sess., 1950, 96, pt. 5:5812.
34. Mrs. Hobby surely would have preferred to control her Department, its programs, and its budgets, but she gave no indication of being willing to fight over the matter. In 1954, in connection with the Administration budget request for $60 million for the Hill-Burton hospital program, Congressman Fogarty asked Secretary Hobby: "What would you say if Congress decided to appropriate three times that amount, or $180 million, for this program?" She replied: "Well, Sir, you know I would never say anything." Fogarty: "I mean do you think the money could be well spent?" *House Appropriations Hearings, 1955*, 84th Cong., 1st sess., "Department of Health, Education and Welfare," pt. 1:115.
35. *Ibid.*, p. 98.
36. *Ibid.*, "Public Health Service," pp. 780–781.
37. *House Appropriations Hearings, 1955*, 83rd Cong., 2nd sess., p. 210.
38. This and 10 succeeding paragraphs are based largely on an interview with Mr. Folsom, 23 Jan. 1970.
39. *Ibid.* Folsom took care of the largest increase, that of classroom construction, differently. He was apparently one Cabinet member on quite good terms with the President's major domo, Sherman Adams; he went to Adams to outline the problem and obtain a judgment about whether this was a matter to be taken up directly with the President. Adams, probably more protective of the President in that period than ever and utterly confident of his own authority, said the matter could be taken care of without bothering the President. With Folsom still in the room, he phoned the Budget Director. His message to Brundage was brief: "This is Adams. You just lost $250 million."
40. *Senate Appropriations Hearings, 1957*, 84th Cong., 2nd sess., "Department of HEW," p. 300.
41. *Ibid.*, p. 307.
42. *Ibid.*
43. *Ibid.*, pp. 508–509.
44. *Senate Committee Report on Labor-Hew Appropriations, 1957*, 84th Cong., 2nd sess., p. 17.

1. *House Appropriations Hearings, 1955*, 83rd Cong., 2nd sess., "Public Health Service," p. 97.
2. *Ibid.*
3. *Senate Committee Report on Labor-HEW Appropriations, 1954*, 84th Cong., 1st sess., p. 19.
4. E.g., see *House Appropriations Hearings, 1958*, 85th Cong., 1st sess., "Public Health Service," p. 995.
5. E.g., *ibid., 1959*, 85th Cong., 2nd sess., "Public Health Service," pp. 470–471.
6. *Ibid., 1956*, 84th Cong., 1st sess., "Department of Health, Education and Welfare," pp. 15, 226–227; "Public Health Service," p. 576.
7. E.g., *ibid., 1960*, 86th Cong., 1st sess., "Public Health Service," p. 879.
8. *Ibid.*, p. 260.
9. *House Appropriations Hearings, 1959*, 85th Cong., 2nd sess., "Public Health Service," pp. 470–471.
10. *Senate Appropriations Hearings, 1958*, 85th Cong., 1st sess., "Public Health Service," p. 1436–1439. The Hill-Humphrey cooperation is interesting, though not surprising to anyone who knows the two, because it was Humphrey's civil rights speech at the Philadelphia convention a decade earlier that had just as dramatically marked the beginning of Lister Hill's decline as of Hubert Humphrey's rise in leadership of the Democratic party.
11. *House Appropriations Hearings, 1958*, 85th Cong., 1st sess., "Public Health Service," p. 420.
12. *Ibid., 1961*, 86th Cong., 2nd sess., "Public Health Service," p. 4.
13. *Ibid.*, pp. 508–509.
14. *Ibid.*, p. 509.
15. *Senate Appropriations Hearings, 1959*, 86th Cong., 2nd sess., "Public Health Service," pp. 1512–1513.
16. Interviews with Dr. Shannon, April 1970, and Dr. Endicott, 10 Nov. 1971.
17. Interview with Dr. Endicott, 10 Nov. 1971.
18. *Senate Committee Report on Labor-HEW Appropriations, 1959*, 85th Cong., 2nd sess., p. 23.
19. *House Appropriations Hearings, 1960*, 86th Cong., 1st sess., "Public Health Service," pp. 415, 418–419.
20. *Ibid., 1958*, 85th Cong., 1st sess., "Public Health Service," p. 422.
21. *Ibid.*, "Testimony of Interested Individuals," pp. 63–64.
22. *Congressional Record*, 84th Cong., 2nd sess., 1956, 102, pt. 4:56771.
23. *Senate Committee Report on Labor-HEW Appropriations, 1962*, 87th Cong., 1st sess., p. 23.
24. *Senate Appropriations Hearings, 1957*, 84th Cong., 2nd sess., p. 733.
25. *Ibid.*
26. *House Appropriations Hearings, 1957*, 85th Cong., 1st sess., "Public Health Service," p. 532.
27. *Senate Appropriations Hearings, 1961*, 86th Cong., 2nd sess., "Public Health Service," p. 554.
28. *Ibid., 1962*, 87th Cong., 1st sess., "Public Health Service," p. 1106.

29. *Ibid., 1959*, 85th Cong., 2nd sess., "Interested Individuals," p. 1506.

30. See, e.g., *Congressional Record*, House, 4 May 1965 (daily ed.), p. 9063.

31. *Senate Appropriations Hearings, 1957*, 84th Cong., 2nd sess., "Public Health Service," p. 587.

32. *Congressional Record*, 85th Cong., 1st sess., 1957, 103, pt. 2:1529.

33. *Ibid.*, 86th Cong., 2nd sess., 1960, 106, pt. 5:6835.

34. *Ibid.*, 84th Cong., 2nd sess., 1956, 102, pt. 3:3940.

35. *Washington Post*, 23 Nov. 1965, p. C6.

36. Interview with Sen. Hruska, 23 Aug. 1965.

37. *Congressional Record*, 83rd Cong., 2nd sess., 1954, 100, pt. 6:8006–8007.

38. *Ibid.*, 87th Cong., 2nd sess., 1962, 108, pt. 10:13949.

39. *Ibid.*, 85th Cong., 1st sess., 1957, 103, pt. 4:5520.

40. *Ibid.*, p. 4414.

41. Interview with Mr. Folsom, 23 Jan. 1970.

42. *House Appropriations Hearings, 1960*, 86th Cong., 1st sess., "Department of Health, Education and Welfare," p. 7.

43. *Ibid.* In an interview in August 1965, Fogarty expressed no quarrel with the Budget Bureau, whose staff he generally thought to be competent and thorough, except that: a) it was so small that it could not cover every aspect of every government program and b) when the President arbitrarily set departmental budget ceilings, BOB in turn arbitrarily set ceilings for given activities, including medical research. But on other occasions, Fogarty evidenced deep, personal hostility toward the Bureau. In 1958 at Secretary Folsom's farewell party, upon introduction to a high-ranking Bureau official whom he had not known before, he rankled when told the man was with the Bureau. Like most of the guests, Fogarty had had a couple of drinks; whether that explains his reaction is not certain. "Where did you say you were from?" he asked, declining the official's proffered handshake. When the agency's name was repeated, Fogarty got red in the face and said: "I want you to know I don't care shit about the Budget Bureau." He repeated the statement three times, each time a little louder. Secretary of Labor James Mitchell and Assistant Secretary of HEW Elliot Richardson grabbed Fogarty by both arms and escorted him out. Meanwhile all conversation stopped, even President Eisenhower looked around to see what the commotion was, and the stunned Bureau official was retrieved from a mild state of shock by a thoughtful Vice President Nixon, who came over and engaged him in conversation. Fogarty's attitude no doubt had mellowed in the intervening years.

Lister Hill says the Bureau was of no consequence in determining medical research policy; he wasn't interested in the Bureau, let alone impressed with it, and says he doesn't even know how it functions. The only thing he did know was that the Bureau didn't appear before his committee; hence, whatever its judgments or rationales, they were of no help to him. Clearly he thought BOB was unimportant.

44. *Congressional Record*, 87th Cong., 2nd sess., 1962, 108, pt. 11:15457.

45. *Ibid.*, 1st sess., 1961, 107, pt. 6:8250–8251.

46. *House Appropriations Hearings, 1958*, 85th Cong., 1st sess., "Public Health Service," p. 898.

47. *Senate Appropriations Hearings, 1961*, 87th Cong., 1st sess., "Public Health Service," p. 1429.
48. *Congressional Record*, 86th Cong., 2nd sess., 1960, 106, pt. 5:6830.
49. *Senate Committee Report on Labor-HEW Appropriations, 1960*, 86th Cong., 1st sess., p. 19.
50. *Congressional Record*, 87th Cong., 2nd sess., 1962, 108, pt. 4:5150.
51. *Senate Appropriations Hearings, 1960*, 86th Cong., 1st sess., "Public Health Service," p. 1221.

Chapter VII. Lobbying Medical Professionals and Professional Medical Lobbyists

1. *House Appropriations Hearings, 1958*, 85th Cong., 1st sess., "Individual Witnesses" (testimony of Dr. Paul Dudley White), p. 11.
2. Interview with Dr. Scheele, 12 Feb. 1970.
3. *House Appropriations Hearings, 1951*, 81st Cong., 2nd sess., "Public Health Service," p. 127.
4. *Senate Appropriations Hearings, 1961*, 86th Cong., 2nd sess., "Public Health Service," p. 1368.
5. See, e.g., *Facts on the Major Killing and Crippling Diseases in the U.S. Today* (New York: National Health Education Committee, 1966).
6. Interviews with Mrs. Mahoney, 1965–1971. See also Elizabeth Drew, "The Health Syndicate: Washington's Nobel Conspirators," *Atlantic Monthly*, December 1967.
7. *House Appropriations Hearings, 1952*, 82nd Cong., 1st sess., "Public Health Service," p. 922.
8. Drew, "The Health Syndicate," p. 77.
9. Interview with Senator Hill, 23 Aug. 1965.
10. *Senate Appropriations Hearings, 1950*, 81st Cong., 1st sess., "Members of Congress, Interest Organizations and Individual Witnesses."
11. *House Appropriations Hearings, 1957*, 85th Cong., 1st sess., "Interested Individual Witnesses," p. 111.
12. *Senate Appropriations Hearings, 1950*, 81st Cong., 1st sess., "Members of Congress, Organizations and Interested Individuals."
13. E.g., see *Senate Appropriations Hearings, 1960*, 86th Cong., 1st sess., "Public Health Service," p. 1221; or *House Appropriations Hearings, 1958*, 85th Cong., 1st sess., "Public Health Service," p. 1482.
14. *Congressional Record*, 83rd Cong., 2nd sess., 1952, 98, pt. 3:2841.
15. *House Appropriations Hearings, 1955*, 83rd Cong., 2nd sess., "Public Health Service," p. 428.
16. *Congressional Record*, 4 May 1965 (daily ed.), p. 9047.
17. *Ibid.* M.D.'s in the House included Congressman Durwood Gorham Hall (R., Mo.), who, despite his reputation for conservatism in every area, that year (1965) strongly supported the Labor-HEW subcommittee report and requested higher budget figures for NIH (*ibid.*, p. 9049).
18. *Senate Appropriations Hearings, 1956*, 84th Cong., 1st sess., "Public Health Service," p. 854.
19. *House Appropriations Hearings, 1959*, 85th Cong., 2nd sess., "Interested Individuals," p. 70.
20. *Ibid.*, 1960, 86th Cong., 1st sess., "Public Health Service," p. 419.

21. *Senate Appropriations Hearings, 1958*, 85th Cong., 1st sess., "Public Health Service," p. 1141.

22. *House Appropriations Hearings, 1959*, 85th Cong., 2nd sess., "Interested Individuals," p. 51.

23. Interview with Dr. Shannon, 23 Sept. 1965.

24. Drew, "The Health Syndicate," p. 79.

25. *Ibid.*

26. *Senate Appropriations Hearings, 1961*, 86th Cong., 2nd sess., "Public Health Service," p. 1388.

27. *House Appropriations Hearings, 1959*, 85th Cong., 2nd sess., "Interested Individuals," p. 106.

28. *Ibid.*, *1957*, 84th Cong., 2nd sess., "Interested Individuals," p. 26.

29. *Ibid.*, *1955*, 83rd Cong., 2nd sess., "Interested Individuals," p. 314.

30. *Ibid.*, *1959*, 85th Cong., 2nd sess., "Interested Individuals," p. 80.

31. *Senate Appropriations Hearings, 1958*, 85th Cong., 2nd sess., "Individual Witnesses," pp. 1447–1448.

32. *Ibid.*, *1959*, 85th Cong., 2nd sess., "Interested Individuals," p. 1506.

33. *House Appropriations Hearings, 1955*, 83rd Cong., 2nd sess., "Interested Individuals," p. 154.

34. *Senate Appropriations Hearings, 1962*, 87th Cong., 1st sess., "Interested Individuals," p. 1106.

35. *House Appropriations Hearings, 1955*, 83rd Cong., 2nd sess., "Interested Individuals," p. 154.

36. *Congressional Record*, 86th Con., 2nd sess., 1960, 106, pt. 10: 13089.

37. *House Appropriations Hearings, 1955*, 83rd Cong., 2nd sess., "Interested Individuals," pp. 210–212.

38. Interview with Dr. Farber, 24 Jan. 1970.

39. *Ibid.*

40. Drew, "The Health Syndicate," p. 78.

41. Mary Lasker had discovered very early that one of the roles she would have to play would be that of messenger. Rather than negotiate directly with his sometime counterpart Styles Bridges for Bridges' support, Hill would ask Mrs. Lasker to go see her friend to feel him out on various propositions. She would, armed with the latest medicine for his hypertension, and more often than not she would get his agreement.

42. Interview with Colonel Quinn, 10 Feb. 1970.

43. E.g., *Congressional Record*, 86th Cong., 2nd sess., 1960, 106, pt. 5:6834–6835.

44. Illustrating Farber's "romantic view of how things happen," Quinn says that the central reason for Ike's decision not to veto the 1961 HEW appropriations bill, with its big increases for NIH, was that Congressman Laird had advised the President that the veto would not be sustained.

45. *House Appropriations Hearings, 1960*, 86th Cong., 1st sess., "Interested Individuals," p. 879.

46. Charles E. Lindblom, *The Policy Making Process* (Englewood Cliffs, N.J.: Prentice-Hall, 1968), p. 65.

47. One of the few persons who consistently appeared before the committees to testify specifically for biomedical science and scientific-educational institutions was Dr. Philip Handler, chairman of the Department of Biochemistry at Duke University, later president of the National Acad-

emy of Sciences. See, e.g., *House Appropriations Hearings, 1963,* 87th Cong., 2nd sess., "Interested Individuals," pp. 165ff.

48. *Report of the Commission on Research* (Chicago: American Medical Association, February 1967).

49. James Z. Appel, "The Practitioners and Health Care," White House Conference on Health, 4 Nov. 1965, p. 7.

50. *Report of the Commission on Research* (AMA), pp. 1–2.

51. *Senate Appropriations Hearings, 1959,* 85th Con., 2nd sess., "Interested Individuals," p. 1671.

52. *Ibid.,* p. 1683.

Chapter VIII. The Dangers of Political Success

1. Interview with Mr. Carey, 30 March 1970.

2. Based on interviews with persons concerned.

3. *The Advancement of Medical Research and Education through the Department of Health, Education and Welfare,* Final Report of the Secretary's Consultants on Medical Research and Education (the Bayne-Jones Report), (Washington: Department of HEW, 1958).

4. *Congressional Record,* 86th Cong., 1st sess., 1959, 105, pt. 9:11730.

5. U.S., Congress, Senate, Committee on Appropriations, *Federal Support of Medical Research,* Report of the Committee of Consultants on Medical Research to the Health Subcommittee (the Jones Report), 86th Cong., 2nd sess., May 1960, p. xii.

6. Interview with Mr. Jones, 2 June 1970. Jones' name had been suggested to Senator Hill by Dr. Ernest M. Allen, longtime official of the Public Health Service and, with Jones, an Emory University alumnus.

7. Elizabeth Drew, "The Health Syndicate," *Atlantic Monthly,* December 1967, p. 76.

8. Charles Lindblom, *The Policy Making Process* (Englewood Cliffs, N.J.: Prentice-Hall, 1968), p. 65.

9. Jones Report, pp. v, xiii, xiv.

10. *Ibid.,* p. xxii.

11. *Senate Committee Report on Labor-HEW Appropriations, 1961,* 86th Cong., 2nd sess., 14 June 1960, p. 18.

12. *Congressional Record,* 87th Cong., 1st sess., 1961, 107, pt. 6:8251.

13. *House Committee Report on Labor-HEW Appropriations, 1962,* 87th Cong., 1st sess., p. 20.

14. *Congressional Record,* 87th Cong., 1st sess., 1961, 107, pt. 14:18822, 19079.

15. *Ibid.,* p. 18822.

16. *Ibid.,* pt. 11:14218.

17. *Ibid.,* 84th Cong., 1st sess., 1955, 101, pt. 6:7627–7628.

18. *Ibid.,* 87th Cong., 2nd sess., 1963, 109, pt. 6:7407.

19. *Ibid.,* p. 7412.

20. *Ibid.,* 88th Cong., 1st sess., 1963, 109, pt. 11:14478.

21. *Ibid.,* pp. 14240, 14475.

22. *Ibid.,* p. 14467.

23. *Ibid.,* 87th Cong., 1st sess., 1961, 107, pt. 11:14248.

24. *Ibid.,* 88th Cong., 1st sess., 1963, 109, pt. 6:7419.

25. E.g., *Congressional Record*, 86th Cong., 2nd sess., 1960, 106, pt. 10:13087; and *ibid.*, 88th Cong., 1st sess., 1963, 109, pt. 11:14496.

26. *Congressional Record*, 86th Cong., 2nd sess., 1960, 106, pt. 10: 13088.

27. *Congressional Record*, 5 Aug. 1965 (daily ed.), p. 18867.

28. *NIH Almanac, 1969* (Bethesda, Md.: NIH Office of Information), p. 91; *Resources for Medical Research*, report no. 10, U.S. Public Health Service, Department of HEW, January 1967, p. 24.

29. U.S., Congress, House, Committee on Government Operations, "The Administration of Grants by the National Institutes of Health," (Fountain Committee hearings), 87th Con., 1st sess., August 1971, p. 110.

30. *Ibid.*, pp. 128, 130.

31. *Ibid.*, pp. 127–128.

32. *Administration of Grants by NIH: Re-examination of Management Deficiencies,* Report of the Fountain Committee, 87th Cong., 2nd sess., 30 June 1962, pp. 3–7.

33. *Ibid.*, pp. 8–9.

34. *Congressional Record*, 87th Cong., 1st sess., 1961, 107, pt. 6:8256.

35. Fountain Committee hearings, March 1962, p. 128.

36. *Ibid.*, p. 14.

37. E.g., interview with Senator Margaret Chase Smith, 1 Sept. 1965.

38. One exception was when Senator Douglas let slip one year, in his attack on the subcommittee's proposed increases, his displeasure with NIH for its treatment of his friend Dr. Ivey, discoverer of the alleged cancer cure Krebiozen. Hill ignored Douglas' fiscal arguments and said: "I am sorry the Senator is disappointed over the results of his efforts in behalf of Krebiozen." *Congressional Record*, 82nd Cong., 2nd sess., 1962, 108, pt. 11:4294.

39. Joseph D. Cooper, "Acute Political Impatience Maintains Pressure on NIH," *Medical Tribune,* 9 Dec. 1968, pp. 7–8.

40. Fountain Committee report, June 1962, p. 25. Dr. Delphis Goldberg, the staff member who directed the inquiry, confirms the significance of Dr. Shannon's response. Goldberg had had some difficulty in getting anybody but Chairman Fountain interested in the probe, and had thought the Committee's investigation might have to be terminated. But Shannon's "arrogance" so offended the members of thet Committee (including Congressmen Neal Smith [D., Iowa], subsequently a member of the Labor-HEW appropriations subcommittee, and Odin Langen [R., Minn.]) that the hearings and the investigation took on new life. Shannon, in turn, was reportedly furious with his staff for not warning him how serious and potentially dangerous the Fountain probe was.

41. *Ibid.*, p. 26.

42. *Biomedical Science and Its Administration* (Woolridge Report), the White House, February 1965, p. xv.

43. *Science,* 11 June 1965, p. 1433.

44. Woolridge Report, p. xv.

45. *Ibid.*

46. *Ibid.*, p. 1. Dr. Cooper, among others, raised questions about various aspects of the Committee's approach and findings. Pointing to the assessment of current research as being of good quality, but suggesting that NIH management capability needed improvement, Cooper asked: "If the

quality of management has been deficient both within NIH and the universities and if, nevertheless, research continues to be of high quality, why be concerned about good management other than to make sure that no funds are improperly diverted? On the other hand, it might be more realistic to ask whether there *can* be a consistently high level of research quality in the face of inadequate management." *Science,* 11 June 1965, p. 1435.

47. Woolridge Report, pp. 2–3.

48. *Congressional Record,* House, 4 May 1965 (daily ed.), 89th Cong., 1st sess., p. 9046.

49. *Congressional Record,* Senate, 5 Aug. 1965 (daily ed.), 89th Cong., 1st sess., p. 18868.

50. Woolridge Report, p. 7.

51. *Congressional Record,* Senate, 5 Aug. 1965 (daily ed.), 89th Cong., 1st sess., p. 18869.

52. *Ibid.,* p. 18861.

53. *Ibid.,* p. 18867.

54. *Ibid.,* p. 18871.

55. Mrs. Lasker had begun cultivating Senator Johnson's interest years before. See Drew, "The Health Syndicate," pp. 76–78.

56. Interview with Congressman Fogarty, 10 Aug. 1965.

Chapter IX. The Breakdown of the Coalition

1. Milton Viorst, "The Political Good Fortune of Medical Research," *Science,* 17 April 1964.

2. See, e.g., "Moving Force in Medical Research," *Medical World News,* 20 Nov. 1964, pp. 83–89.

3. Elizabeth Drew, "The Health Syndicate," *Atlantic Monthly,* December 1967, p. 78.

4. "Moving Force in Medical Research," p. 84.

5. *Ibid.*

6. James A. Shannon, M.D., "The Advancement of Medical Research: A Twenty-Year View of the NIH Role," Alan Gregg Memorial Lecture, San Francisco, 22 Oct. 1966.

7. *Ibid.,* p. 19.

8. Senator Hill commented during the hearings in 1956: "My mind continually goes to the atomic bomb. If we had sat down and said, 'Well now, we can't spend too much . . . we have to take this a little more slowly,' we wouldn't have gotten the bomb when we did." *Senate Appropriations Hearings, 1957,* 84th Cong., 2nd sess., "Interested Individuals," p. 1054. He continued to want results, but he dropped that particular comparison as time went on.

9. *Senate Committee Report on Labor-HEW Appropriations, 1967,* 90th Cong., 1st sess.

10. *Congressional Record,* 86th Cong., 1st sess., 1959, 105, pt. 9:11722.

11. *House Appropriations Hearings, 1956,* 84th Cong., 2nd sess., "Public Health Service," p. 538.

12. Omnibus Medical Research Act of 1950, 64 *Stat.* 443 (P.L. 81-692).

13. Drew, "The Health Syndicate," p. 81.

14. Language of the Ransdell Act, which reorganized, expanded, and redesignated the Hygienic Laboratory as the National Institutes of Health (46 Stat. 585 [P.L. 71-357]).

15. As quoted by Dr. Kenneth M. Endicott, interview 2 Dec. 1970.

16. *House Committee Report on Labor-HEW Appropriations, 1966,* 89th Cong., 1st sess., p. 36.

17. *House Committee Report, 1963,* 87th Con., 2nd sess., p. 38.

18. *Senate Committee Report, 1957,* 85th Con., 1st sess., p. 18.

19. *House Committee Report, 1962,* 87th Cong., 1st sess., p. 29.

20. Interview with Dr. Shannon, 23 Sept. 1965. Some such directives were put into the reports at the request of the NIH managers, to give them specific support, if not specific reason, for engaging in given activities or doing things a certain way. Some, however, originated with the committees and were inserted despite the reservations or objections of NIH officials.

21. *Senate Committee Report for Labor-HEW Appropriations, 1962,* 87th Cong., 1st sess., pp. 27–28.

22. *House Appropriations Hearings, 1963,* 88th Cong., 1st sess., "Interested Individuals," p. 398.

23. U.S., Congress, House, Committee on Government Operations, "Hearings on the Administration of Grants by NIH" (Fountain Committee hearings), 87th Cong., 2nd sess., March 1962, pp. 109–110.

24. *Ibid.*

25. *Senate Committee Report on Labor-HEW Appropriations, 1961,* 86th Cong., 2nd sess., p. 31.

26. *Biomedical Science and Its Administration* (Woolridge Report), the White House, February 1965, pp. 42–43.

27. *House Committee Report on Labor-HEW Appropriations, 1960,* 86th Cong., 1st sess., pp. 17–18.

28. Drew, "The Health Syndicate," p. 80.

29. Interview with Dr. Farber, 24 Jan. 1970.

30. Interview with Dr. Rusk, 17 Dec. 1969.

31. Joseph D. Cooper, "Health, Research, and Goals Pose Guidelines Problems for NIH" (part of a series), *Medical Tribune,* 16 Dec. 1968, p. 1.

32. *Ibid.*

33. *Senate Appropriations Hearings, 1957,* 84th Cong., 2nd sess., "Interested Individuals," p. 1341.

34. Interview with Col. Luke Quinn, 10 Feb. 1970.

35. Interview with Dr. DeBakey, 4 March 1970. See also Drew, "The Health Syndicate," pp. 79–80.

36. *Senate Committee Report on Labor-HEW Appropriations, 1964,* 88th Cong., 1st sess., p. 48.

37. *Report of the Secretary's Advisory Committee on the Management of NIH Research Grants and Contracts* (Ruina Report), Department of HEW, March 1966, esp. pp. 1–2.

38. Ruina Report, p. 31.

39. Interview with Dr. Shannon, 29 April 1970.

40. Fountain Committee hearings, March 1964, p. 111.

41. Drew, "The Health Syndicate," p. 76.

42. *Ibid.,* p. 80.

43. *New York Times,* 28 June 1966, p. 1.

44. Drew, "The Health Syndicate," p. 81.

45. *House Appropriations Hearings, 1960,* 86th Cong., 1st sess., "Interested Individuals" (testimony of Dr. Walter Bauer, Massachusetts General Hospital), p. 120.

46. John W. Gardner, "The Government, the Universities, and Biomedical Research," *Science,* 30 Sept. 1966, pp. 1602–1603.

47. Drew, "The Health Syndicate," p. 81.

48. Interview with Mr. Cater, 29 May 1970.

Chapter X. The End of an Era

1. See hearings and reports (nos. 1–10) of the Select Committee on Government Research, U.S. House of Representatives, 88th Congress, 1st and 2nd sess., 1963–1965.

2. Carey, "Research and Development and the Federal Budget," 17th National Conference on Administration of Research, Estes Park, Col., 11 Sept. 1963.

3. Quoted in Joseph D. Cooper, "A Time of Crisis for NIH" (1st article in a series), *Medical Tribune,* 28 Nov. 1968, p. 2.

4. Joseph D. Cooper, "Clearer Goals and Priorities Hold Keys for Future of NIH," *Medical Tribune,* 6 Jan. 1969, p. 19.

5. *House Appropriations Hearings, 1963,* 88th Cong., 1st sess., letter from Dr. Shannon to Congressman Fogarty transmitting projections of national medical research expenditures for five years, p. iii.

6. *House Appropriations Hearings, 1960,* 86th Con., 2nd sess., "Public Health Service," p. 137.

7. 77 *Stat.* 164 (P.L. 88-129).

8. Social Security Amendments of 1965, 79 *Stat.* 286 (P.L. 89-97), Titles 1, 2.

9. U.S., Congress, House, Committee on Government Operations, *Hearings on Health Research and Training* (Fountain Committee hearings), 87th Cong., 1st sess., August 1961, p. 83.

10. *Washington Post,* 3 Sept. 1967, pp. 7, A5. A report in the *British Medical Journal,* 23 December 1971, on a five-year study in England indicates that Atromid (clofibrate) can be an effective control agent for patients with ischaemic heart disease. The British study began at about the time the American study would have begun, if Mrs. Lasker had prevailed.

11. Fountain Committee report, Oct., 1967. The exception was for fiscal 1964, when the budget estimate for NIH was $742 million, the House voted $736 million, the Senate voted $741 million, and the final appropriation that the House insisted upon was $736 million.

12. *Washington Post,* 22 Oct. 1967, p. A6.

13. *Science,* 3 Nov. 1967.

14. *Ibid.,* pp. 613–614.

15. *Ibid.,* p. 611.

16. *Washington Post,* 22 Oct. 1967, p. A6.

17. Joseph D. Cooper, "NIH Appraisals Are Difficult," *Medical Tribune,* 19 Dec. 1968, p. 11.

18. *Science,* 26 Dec. 1969, editorial page.

19. These figures, and trends, are seen most easily in the summary table of NIH appropriations and obligations, *House Appropriations Hearings, 1971,* 91st Cong., 2nd sess., "National Institutes of Health," p. 50. The National Institute of Mental Health, with its extensive state services program, was pulled out of NIH in 1967 and made a separate bureau within the Public Health Service. With an annual budget of over $200 million per year for the last three fiscal years of the decade, its removal from NIH made the medical research agency's budget seem even more retarded in growth. The House Appropriations Subcommittee revised its figures in the "Appropriations History and Obligations, 1961–71" after the reorganization, so NIH budgets, appropriations, and obligations from 1961 do not include NIMH for any years. The meaning of all this is simply that, including the Mental Health Institute's budget, NIH reached the $1-billion-plus appropriation level in fiscal 1966 (1965); minus NIMH, NIH went over the $1 billion mark in appropriations a year later (*ibid.,* pp. 48–49).

20. Elizabeth Drew, "The Health Syndicate," *Atlantic Monthly,* December 1967, p. 82.

21. *Congressional Record,* 83rd Cong., 2nd sess., 1954, 100, pt. 6:7965.

22. *Ibid.,* 85th Cong., 1st sess., 1957, 103, pt. 4:4409.

23. Conversation with Congressman Mahon, March 1971.

24. *Congressional Record,* 88th Cong., 1st sess., 1963, 109, pt. 11:14498.

25. "Moving Force in Medical Research," *Medical World News,* 20 Nov. 1964, p. 85.

26. Drew, "The Health Syndicate," p. 81.

27. "Moving Force in Medical Research," *Medical World News,* p. 83.

28. *Ibid.,* p. 84.

29. Interview with Dr. Shannon, 23 Sept. 1965.

30. *Ibid.,* 29 April 1970.

31. Interview with Mrs. Lasker, 13 Jan. 1970.

32. "Moving Force in Medical Research," *Medical World News,* p. 89. As for important agency figures in the Cause, former Director of NIH Rolla E. Dyer, and former NIH Deputy Director C. J. Van Slyke, are among those who have received the Lasker awards. Dr. Shannon is not.

33. Interview with Mrs. Lasker, 17 Oct. 1971.

34. Interviews with Senator Hill, 30 Aug. 1965, 26 Nov. 1969.

35. Interview with Congressman Fogarty, 10 Aug. 1965.

36. *Congressional Record,* 87th Cong., 2nd sess., 1962, 108, pt. 11:5161.

37. *Ibid.,* 88th Cong., 1st sess., 1963, 109, pt. 6:7149.

38. *Congressional Record,* House, 21 July 1970 (daily ed.), p. 6991.

39. *Senate Appropriations Hearings, 1970,* 91st Cong., 1st sess., "National Institutes of Health," p. 1017.

40. *Ibid., 1957,* 85th Cong., 1st sess., "Interested Individuals," p. 1374.

41. *Science,* 26 Dec. 1969, editorial page.

Chapter XI. An Assessment of Policy Results

1. Daniel S. Greenberg, *The Politics of Pure Science* (New York: New American Library, 1967), p. 200.

2. *Senate Committee Report on Labor-Federal Security Appropriations,* *1950*, 81st Cong., 1st sess., p. 16.

3. *Senate Committee Report on Labor-HEW Appropriations, 1950,* 86th Cong., 2nd sess., pp. 19–20.

4. *House Appropriations Hearings, 1962,* 87th Cong., 2nd sess., "Public Health Service," p. 408.

5. *Biomedical Science and Its Administration* (Woolridge Report), the White House, February 1965, pp. 2, 3.

6. *Ibid.*

7. Cooper, "Onward the Management of Science: The Woolridge Report," *Science,* 11 June 1965, p. 1344.

8. Cooper, "Time of Crisis for NIH," *Medical Tribune,* 28 Nov. 1968.

9. *Report of the Commission on Research* (Whittaker Commission), American Medical Association, February 1967, p. 6.

10. *Journal of Medical Education,* 45, no. 4 (April 1970), 250.

11. *Federal Support for Medical Research,* Report of the Committee on Consultants to the Senate Appropriations Subcommittee on Labor-HEW Appropriations (Jones Committee), 86th Cong., 2nd sess., May 1960, p. xv.

12. Whittaker Commission report, pp. 38, 39.

13. Stephen P. Strickland, ed., *Population Crisis: A Condensation of U.S. Senate Hearings* (Washington: Socio-Dynamics Publications, 1970), p. 321.

14. Elizabeth Drew, "The Health Syndicate," *Atlantic Monthly,* December 1967, p. 82.

15. Editorial, *Medical World News,* 30 Jan. 1970, p. 52.

16. *Ibid.*

17. *What Should Be the Level of Support for Biomedical Research During the Next Five Years,* Issue Paper prepared by the Office of the Associate Director for Program Planning and Evaluation, National Institutes of Health, October 1971, app. A, p. 12.

18. *Ibid.,* pp. 13–14.

19. *Progress Against Cancer, 1970,* Report of the National Advisory Cancer Council, U.S. Department of Health, Education and Welfare (Public Health Service, National Institutes of Health), p. 14.

20. *Highlights in the Scientific History and Organization of the National Institutes of Health* (Bethesda, Md.: NIH Office of Information, Fall 1970), p. 14.

21. *Ibid.,* p. 27.

22. *Ibid.,* p. 28.

23. See, e.g., John A. Osmundsen, "Gene Has Made Its Mark in Medicine This Year," *Washington Post,* 27 Dec. 1970, p. D2.

24. *Washington Post,* 20 Nov. 1970, p. 4.

25. *Washington Evening Star,* 20 Nov. 1970, p. 14.

26. *Washington Post,* 12 Feb. 1970, p. A42.

27. Harvard Medical School's total institutional budget climbed from $3.245 million in 1950 to $28.720 million in 1970, an increase of almost 800 percent. Federal funds, which amounted to 21 percent of the school's budget 20 years ago, now amount to 58 percent of the total; and federal *research* funds (of which NIH funds consistently make up the dominant portion) amount to 41 percent of the total.

Case Western Reserve University Medical School's total budget has grown from $2.2 million in 1950 to $16.4 in 1970, with federal funds amounting to 34 percent of the total then and 59 percent of the total now; research funds made up 30 percent of Case Western's budget in 1950, and today they constitute 40 percent of the total. Baylor Medical College's budget has risen from a little over $700,000 in 1950 to over $21 million in 1970 largely because of federal funds, which have increased from $80,000 in 1950 to $14.8 million in 1970; federal funds amount to about 70 percent of that college's budget at present.

At the Medical College of Alabama, federal funds amount to 80 percent of the institution's total budget of $27.6 million in 1970, up from 50 percent only 12 years ago; NIH funds alone constitute 65 percent of the college's budget this year. At the University of Pennsylvania Medical School, where there is a long tradition of research, federal research funds comprise almost 65 percent of the total institutional budget of $27.9 million this year.

The figures here and in paragraphs relating to medical school budgets and M.D. and Ph.D. enrollments were supplied by the institutions discussed.

28. Jones Committee report, p. xv.

29. Whittaker Commission report, pp. 39–40.

30. U.S., Congress, House, Committee on Interstate and Foreign Commerce, *Hearings on National Health Plan,* 81st Cong., 1st sess., p. 50.

31. U.S., Congress, Senate, Committee on Labor and Public Welfare, *Hearings on National Health Insurance,* 1949, 81st Cong., 1st sess., p. 639.

32. *Ibid.,* pp. 210–211.

33. *Building America's Health,* Report to the President, 18 Dec. 1952 (Washington: Government Printing Office), pp. 13, 20–21.

34. U.S., Department of Health, Education and Welfare, *The Advancement of Medical Research and Education through the Department of HEW,* Report of the Secretary's Consultants on Medical Research and Education, 1958.

35. U.S., Department of Health, Education and Welfare, *Physicians for a Growing America,* Report of the Surgeon General's Consultant Group on Medical Education, 1959.

36. *House Committee Report on Labor-HEW Appropriations, 1958,* 85th Cong., 1st sess., p. 17.

37. 77 *Stat.* 164 (P.L. 88-129).

38. Health Professions Educational Assistance Act of 1963, 79 *Stat.* 164 (P.L. 88-129); Health Professions Act Amendments of 1965, 79 *Stat.* 1050 (P.L. 89-290); Health Manpower Act of 1968, 82 *Stat.* 773 (P.L. 90-490).

39. *The Life Sciences,* Report of the Committee on Research in the Life Sciences, National Academy of Sciences, 1970, p. 307.

40. *NIH Almanac, 1969* (Bethesda, Md.: NIH Office of Information) pp. 81–83. In 1968 the National Institute of Mental Health became a separate bureau; more of its grant funds were invested in training programs than in research. Hence the dollar level and the percentage of training funds (as against research funds) both declined for NIH with that separation of NIMH from the other Institutes.

41. *The Life Sciences*, pp. 306–307.

42. Joseph D. Cooper, "Clearer Goals and Priorities for NIH," *Medical Tribune*, 6 Jan. 1969.

43. P.L. 92-157, 18 Nov. 1971.

44. *Congressional Record* (daily ed.), 25 Jan. 1971, p. 87.

Chapter XII. Conquering Cancer: Renewing the Goal

1. Yarborough, press release, 25 March 1970.

2. *National Journal*, 3, no. 13 (27 March 1971), 678.

3. U.S., Congress, Senate, Committee on Labor and Public Welfare, *National Program for the Conquest of Cancer* (Report of the National Panel of Consultants on the Conquest of Cancer), 91st Cong., 2nd sess., November 1970.

4. *Ibid.*, pt. 1:1.

5. U.S., Congress, House of Representatives, *H. Con. Res. 675*, 91st Cong., 2nd sess., 15 July 1970.

6. *Washington Post*, 5 Dec. 1970, pp. 1, 3.

7. As reported in the *Washington Evening Star*, 23 Jan. 1971, p. A7.

8. *National Journal*, 3, no. 13 (27 March 1971), 678.

9. U.S., Congress, Senate, Senate Bill 34, 92nd Cong., 1st sess., January 1971; see *Hearings of the Senate Labor and Public Welfare Committee on Conquest of Cancer Act, 1971*, pp. 3–19.

10. *Ibid.*, p. 17 of S. 34; p. 19 of Senate hearings.

11. As quoted by Cristine Russell, "The Politics of Cancer," *Washington Post*, 28 Nov. 1971, p. C5.

12. U.S., Congress, Senate, Committee on Labor and Public Welfare, *Hearings on Conquest of Cancer Act, 1971*, 92nd Cong., 1st sess., March and June 1971, pp. 64–68.

13. *Ibid.*, p. 29.

14. *Ibid.*, p. 205.

15. Quoted by Lucy Eisenberg in "The Politics of Cancer," *Harper's Magazine*, November 1971, p. 104.

16. *Conquest of Cancer Act, 1971*, Senate hearings, pp. 265–266.

17. *Ibid.*, p. 25.

18. *National Journal*, 3, no. 13 (27 March 1971), 676.

19. *Ibid.*, 3, no. 31 (31 July 1971), 1616.

20. *Conquest of Cancer Act, 1971*, Senate hearings, pp. 121–123.

21. *Ibid.*, p. 89.

22. *Washington Post*, 20 April 1971, p. B5.

23. *National Journal*, 3, no. 31 (21 July 1971), 1615.

24. *Conquest of Cancer Act, 1971*, Senate hearings, p. 202.

25. Interview with Mr. Cole, 4 Oct. 1971.

26. *Ibid.*

27. *Washington Post*, 12 May 1971, p. 1.

28. *Conquest of Cancer Act, 1971*, Senate hearings, pp. 298–304.

29. *National Journal*, 3, no. 31 (31 July 1971), 1611.

30. *Ibid.*, p. 1612.

31. Interview with Dr. DuVal, 8 Nov. 1971.

32. *Conquest of Cancer Act, 1971*, Senate hearings, pp. 372–373.

33. U.S., Congress, House of Representatives, Committee on Interstate and Foreign Commerce, *Hearings on National Cancer Attack Act of 1971,* 92nd Cong., 1st sess., pt. 2:648.

34. See, e.g., *National Journal,* 3, no. 103 (27 March 1971), 680; *Washington Post,* 10 December 1971.

35. *Conquest of Cancer Act, 1971,* Senate hearings, p. 112.

36. U.S., Congress, *Congressional Record* (daily ed.), 92nd Cong., 1st sess., 19 July 1971, pp. H6882–6883.

37. U.S., Congress, House of Representatives, Committee on Interstate and Foreign Commerce, *Investigation of HEW,* Report of the Special Subcommittee on Investigation of the Department of Health, Education and Welfare, 89th Cong., 2nd sess., pp. 107–132.

38. U.S., Congress, House of Representatives, Committee on Interstate and Foreign Commerce, *Hearings on National Cancer Attack Act of 1971,* 92nd Cong., 1st sess., vols. 1, 2.

39. P.L. 92-157, 18 Nov. 1971 (the Comprehensive Health Manpower Training Act of 1971).

40. See, e.g., *Washington Post,* 12 Oct. 1971, p. A15.

41. Ronald Sarro, "Cancer Agency Issue: Society Denies It Lobbies," *Washington Star,* 15 Oct. 1971.

42. *National Cancer Attack Act of 1971,* House hearings, pt. 1:143–144.

43. U.S., Congress, *Congressional Record* (daily ed.), 15 Nov. 1971, 92nd Cong., 1st sess., p. 1101.

44. *Ibid.,* pp. 11012–11013.

45. The conference was marked by the unusual but not unique circumstance that the chairman of the House conferees, Congressman Staggers, actually favored the Senate position, while several members of the Senate conference committee would rather have switched to the House version than fight for the one they had first embraced.

46. P.L. 92-157, 18 Nov. 1971.

47. U.S., Congress, *Congressional Record* (daily ed.), 9 Dec. 1971, 92nd Cong., 1st sess., p. H12113.

48. *Ibid.,* 15 Nov. 1971, p. 11015.

49. U.S., the White House, "Statement by the President," 23 Dec. 1971.

50. *Washington Star,* 23 Dec. 1971, p. B5.

51. *Washington Star,* 3 June 1971, p. B4.

52. U.S., the White House, "Statement by the President," 23 Dec. 1971.

53. *Ibid.*

Index

Hinsey, Dean Joseph C., 64–65
Hobby, Mrs. Oveta Culp, 97–98, 101
Hoffman, Anna Rosenberg, 39, 101, 261, 272
Hoover, Herbert, 65
Hoover Commission, 50
Hruska, Sen. Roman, 94, 125, 146
Huggins, Dr. Charles, 149
Humphrey, George, 101, 103, 127, 158
Humphrey, Sen. Hubert H., 68, 72, 113, 126

Institute of Allergy and Infectious Diseases, National, 140, 192, 247
Institute of Arthritis and Metabolic Diseases, 84, 116
Institute of General Medical Sciences, 140
Institute of Neurological Diseases and Blindness, National, 84, 140
Insurance, *see* Health insurance, national
Ives, Sen. Irving, 53

Jackson, Dr. Dudley, 11–12
Javits, Sen. Jacob, 261, 262; and Conquest of Cancer Act (Kennedy-Javits bill), 265, 269–276, 288
Jenner, Edward, 202
Jensen, Rep. Ben Franklin, 121–122, 191
Jewett, Dr. Frank B., 37
Johnson, Dr. Samuel, 143
Johnson, Sen. Hiram, 11
Johnson, Lady Bird (Mrs. Lyndon B.), 206–207
Johnson, Lyndon B., 204, 218, 230, 261; and effect of Vietnam on research budget, 87, 214; and Woolridge Committee, 178; interest of, in health, 181–183; and Mary Lasker, 182, 206–207; support of, for medical research, 191; his challenge to NIH directorate, 207–209; retirement of, 222, 264
Johnston, Eric, 36, 134

Jones, Boisfeullet, 249; Committee of, 160–162, 238, 241
Jones, Dr. T. Duckett, 83
Jones Report, 252
Judd, Rep. Walter, 123

Kaiser, Henry, 42
Kaplan, Dr. Henry S., 270
Keefe, Rep. Frank, 77–82, 88–89, 138
Keefer, Dr. Chester, 17–18
Kennedy, Sen. Edward M., 256, 268, 288; and report of Committee of Consultants, 263; interest of, in health matters, 264; and Conquest of Cancer Act (Kennedy-Javits bill), 265, 269–276; Richardson's letter to, 266–267, 273; his plan merges with Nixon's, 275–276, 280, 282, 285–287; and 1971 Cancer Act, 289
Kennedy-Javits bill, *see* Conquest of Cancer Act
Kennedy, John F., 233, 264; and NIH budget, 162–163, 164–166, 171, 173, 215, 217; asks review of research effort, 177; assassination of, 178, 204
Kennedy, Sen. Robert F., 264
Kerr, Sen. Robert, 68, 69, 72
Kidd, Dr. Charles V., 211
Kidney disease, 242
Kilgore, Sen. Harley, 24, 39, 41
Kingsley, J. Donald, 60–61
Kirwan, Rep. Mike, 153
Kline, Dr. Nathan, 196
Krim, Arthur, 261
Krim, Dr. Mathilde, 261

Ladies Home Journal, 139
LaFollette, Sen. Robert, 14, 46
Laird, Melvin, 114–115, 117, 140, 218; on crash research, 118; and NIH budget, 128–129, 143, 159, 163, 166; and Fountain Comittee, 174; and progress in research, 189–190; on medical research, 213; appointed Secretary of Defense, 222; Fogarty on, 229

Maverick, Mrs. Maury, 12
Medicaid and Medicare, 213–214
Mental Health Division (of PHS), 82, 83
Mental illness, advances in treatment of, 243
Miami Daily News, 33, 46, 137
Michel, Rep. Bob, 231
Miller, Rep. Arthur L. (M.D.), 180–181
Miller, Rep. George, 130
Monaghan, Rep. John, 153
Mountain, Dr. Joe, 44
Multiple Sclerosis Society, 140
Mundt, Sen. Karl, 167
Murray, Sen. James, 53; and Truman's health program, 57, 58; and emergency medical aid bill, 66, 67, 71
Murtagh, Joseph, 270
Muscular Dystrophy Association, 140
Myer, Eugene, 46

National Academy of Sciences, 2–3, 16, 253, 254
National Advisory Council, 53, 135–136; on Health, 114; on Heart, 142; on Cancer, 142–143, 204–205, 265, 289
National Aeronautics and Space Administration, 211
National Cancer Authority, proposed, 262, 265
National Cancer Board, 289
National Cancer Institute, 35, 44, 265, 267, 284; functions of, 14; budget, 49, 83, 134, 260; and chemotherapy program, 200, 204–205, 247; and training grants, 253; and Committee of Consultants, 262; and new cancer plan, 265, 267, 276, 284, 289
National Cancer Institute Act, 13, 24, 245
National Committee for Blinding Eye Diseases and Disability, 140
National Committee on Mental Health, 137, 140

National Committee for Mental Hygiene, 45
National Committee Against Mental Illness, 111, 137–138, 196
National Committee for Research in Neurological Disorders, 140
National Conference on the Problems of Medical Care, 38
National Cystic Fibrosis Association, 140
National Defense Research Committee (NDRC), 15
National Foundation for Infantile Paralysis, 248
National Fund for Medical Education, 65
National Health Education Committee, Inc., 137
National Health Program (1949), Truman's, 57–61, 63, 64, 75
National Health Survey (1936), 33
National Heart Institute, 142, 253; budget, 83; and Atromid-S, 216. *See also* Heart disease
National Heart Institute Act, 53, 95, 135
National Institute(s) of Health: establishment of, 3–4, 25; Conference Board on, 9–10; and wartime research contracts, 26–31; and heart disease, 51–53; becomes National Institutes of Health, 53; as center of medical research empire, 75, 76, 223–224; goals of, contrasted with NSF, 85; and national medical research policy, 86; and policies and politics, 110, 111; and grant proposals, 114–115; members of Congress on, 121–123; expenditures of, 169–170; Fountain Committee study of, 171–174, 176–177, 218–222; Woolridge Committee study of, 177–180; Lyndon Johnson's challenge to, 207–209; and national biomedical science network, 236–240; and effectiveness of disease conquest, 243, 244, 245, 247, 248; and new cancer program, 267–

270, 274–280, 284, 287–289. *See also* Budget, National Institute(s) of Health
National Institute of Mental Health, 112, 129–130, 196, 243, 253
National Medical Research Foundation, proposed, 21, 41
National Mental Health Act, 45
National Science Foundation (NSF), 40, 53; proposed, 19–21, 23, 26; creation of, 84; goals of, contrasted with NIH, 85; and national medical research policy, 86
Neely, Sen. Matthew M., 47, 84, 110, 260, 290; his proposal for cancer research, 1–5, 7–9, 78, 263; new version of his cancer bill, 41, 48; death of, from cancer, 133, 191
Nelson, Rep. Ancher, 285
Nelson, Sen. Gaylord, 270, 276–277, 288
Neuberger, Sen. Richard, 139
New York Times, 38, 94, 202, 246
NIH, *see* National Institute(s) of Health
Nirenberg, Marshall, 239
Nixon, Richard M., 103, 232, 277; his attitude toward medical research, 222, 230; his health plan, 255–256, 258; and NIH budget, 263–264; his cancer plan, 263–264, 265–266, 272–274, 284; his cancer plan merges with Kennedy's, 275–276, 280, 282, 285, 286–287; and Cancer Act of 1971, 288–291
Nixon-Kennedy (-Schmidt-Lasker) bill, 275, 280–287. *See also* Cancer Act of 1971; Conquest of Cancer Act; Kennedy, Edward M.; Nixon, Richard M.
NSF, *see* National Science Foundation

Office of Scientific Research and Development (OSRD), 16, 17, 22; creation of, 15; dissolution of, 29, 30

O'Hara, Rep. Jim, 153
Omnibus Medical Research Act, 84
OSRD, *see* Office of Scientific Research and Development

Palmer, Dr. Walter, 20, 26, 27
Parkinson's disease, 242, 248
Parran, Dr. Thomas, 10, 20, 23, 193; and reorganization of PHS, 18; on cancer institute, 24; on postwar medical research needs, 26; his six-point health program, 46–47; and cancer funds for NIH, 48–49; and heart disease, 51; succeeded by Dr. Scheele, 52, 100
Pastore, Sen. John O., 125, 149, 229; and emergency medical aid bill, 67, 68, 70–71, 72
Penicillin, development of, 16, 17–18
Pepper, Sen. Claude: his subcommittee, 19, 20; and proposed Medical Research Foundation, 21, 41; on medical research, 26–27, 44; his hearings on postwar medical research, 34, 37, 38–39, 40; support of, for Neely bill, 41, 48–49; and Mental Health Act, 44; and heart disease legislation, 51, 53; and Truman's health program, 57; and Taft's health bill, 60; and newly drafted health bill, 62; and Chavez committee, 84; and proposed cancer bill, 286
PHS, *see* Public Health Service
Pickle, Rep. Jake, 285–286
Pneumonia, 241
Potter, Sen. Charles, 106, 122
Priest, Rep. Percy, 44–46
Proximire, Sen. William, 124–125; and NIH budget, 164, 167–169; on Johnson Administration, 181–182
Public Health Service (PHS), 20, 40, 77–78; and cancer research, 4, 8–9, 10–12, 14; reorganization of, 18–19; and policy gap of 1945–46, 23, 26, 27; and Ransdell Act, 25, 26; and wartime re-

Wagner, Sen. Robert, 57
Wagner-Murray-Dingell proposal,
  57–58
Warren, Gov. Earl, 138
Washington Post, 46, 124, 215–
  216, 218
Washington Star, 172
Waterman, Dr. Alan, 85, 212
Weaver, Dr. Harry, 119
Weed, Dr. Lewis, 15, 18
Weinberg, Dr. Alvin, 175
West, Dr. Olin, 14
Wherry, Sen. Kenneth, 133
Whitaker, Clem, 63
White, Dr. Paul Dudley, 83, 104,
  142, 146–147

Whittaker Commission, *see* Amer-
  can Medical Association, Com-
  mission on Research
Williams, Sen. Harrison, 288
Wilson, Mr. and Mrs. Luke I., 11
Wittson, Dr. Cecil, 146, 160
Wolverton, Rep. Charles A., 45,
  122–123, 225
Woolridge (Dr. Dean E.) Com-
  mittee, 177–180, 182, 238–239
Wright, Dr. Irving, 203

Yarborough, Sen. Ralph, 260–262,
  264, 265
Youngdahl, Gov. Luther, 138